OTHER VOLUMES IN
EXERCISES IN DIAGNOSTIC RADIOLOGY

Published

Volume 1 – Squire, Colaiace and Strutynsky: *The Chest*
Volume 2 – Squire, Colaiace and Strutynsky: *The Abdomen*
Volume 3 – Squire, Colaiace and Strutynsky: *Bone*
Volume 5 – Heller and Squire: *Pediatrics*
Volume 6 – James and Squire: *Nuclear Radiology*

Forthcoming

Langston and Squire: *The Emergency Patient*
Squire, Colaiace and Strutynsky: *Special Procedures*

EXERCISES IN DIAGNOSTIC RADIOLOGY

4

THE TOTAL PATIENT

LUCY FRANK SQUIRE, M.D.

Lecturer on Radiology, Harvard Medical School;
Visiting Radiologist, Massachusetts General
Hospital, Boston; Professor in Radiology,
Downstate Medical Center, Brooklyn

JACK R. DREYFUSS, M.D.

Associate Clinical Professor of Radiology,
Harvard Medical School; Radiologist,
Massachusetts General Hospital, Boston

CHARLES S. LANGSTON, M.D.

Instructor in Radiology, Harvard Medical School;
Assistant in Radiology, Massachusetts General
Hospital, Boston

ROBERT A. NOVELLINE, M.D.

Clinical Fellow in Radiology, Harvard Medical
School; Resident in Radiology, Massachusetts
General Hospital, Boston

W. B. SAUNDERS COMPANY • PHILADELPHIA • LONDON • TORONTO

W. B. Saunders Company: West Washington Square
Philadelphia, Pa.   19105

12 Dyott Street
London, WC1A   1DB

833 Oxford Street
Toronto, Ontario M8Z 5T9, Canada

Exercises in Diagnostic Radiology — Volume IV The Total Patient   ISBN 0-7216-8528-5

Print No.:   9   8   7   6   5   4   3

PREFACE FOR
STUDENTS AND TEACHERS

This volume is based on an evening seminar devised for medical students on radiology elective at the Massachusetts General Hospital. We have been giving this seminar since 1967. Its purpose is to afford the students some practice in deciding which radiographic procedures to plan for their patients, in what order, and why.

The students are supplied in advance with a series of short historical vignettes of a dozen or so "patients" who present in the emergency ward or clinic with a variety of both straightforward and complex problems. After having dinner with the radiology teaching staff members, the students in turn choose a "patient," read out the history and outline their proposed management of the case, including what part radiology has in the diagnostic work-up. The other students may agree, disagree, or comment. Finally, the staff members discuss the case.

So many students at MGH have enjoyed this exercise that four of us involved with undergraduate teaching have adapted "the supper seminar" to book form, using actual patients, their medical records, and their x-ray films. Although the clinical data are factual, all names and some of the historical items have been invented.

The book is divided into sequential parts designated by letters, each part adding a little more information about the patients. The Parts are designated for easy thumbing by a dark line on the right margin of each pagespread. The reader should begin with any vignette in Part A and decide how he will manage the patient and what radiology has to offer. The x-rays the student "asks for" are supplied from Part to Part as the story develops. Some situations are intentionally included in which radiographic studies are not needed or are actually contraindicated. The cases are in random order and not intended to follow any sort of progression.

Because we feel so strongly that there can be no isolation of the roentgen investigation from the patient and his medical problems and personal concerns, we have made each case as lifelike and clinically oriented as possible. However, we do not pretend that the medical and radiologic approaches we have used are the only ones to be followed. Although we are grateful to our colleagues in medicine, surgery, and radiology at MGH for their valuable suggestions while we were setting up these cases, we recognize that clinical expediency and local custom often dictate the actual management of any given case. Therefore, students may wish to discuss with their own instructors alternative approaches that might be used to solve these problem cases.

Limitations of size and format have determined the number of cases in the book, but teaching radiologists (or even enterprising students) will be able to set up similar problem-film cases to illustrate additional important and practical points.

We hope that students will enjoy being "on call" to render assistance to the 41 patients in this book—but we hope even more that they will learn some of the ways in which radiology can be of help to them in unraveling the sometimes complex problems presented by the total patient.

LUCY FRANK SQUIRE
JACK R. DREYFUSS
CHARLES S. LANGSTON
ROBERT A. NOVELLINE

Massachusetts General Hospital
Boston, Massachusetts 02114

ACKNOWLEDGMENTS

The need for this kind of exercise was first pointed out to us by a group of fourth year students. To them, and to the many students who have participated in these seminars since, go our warm thanks. Their discussion and their ideas have molded our choice of case-problems, and although a few of the patients included in this book ultimately prove to have uncommon disease conditions, the work-up for that kind of case has been exemplified because the students asked for it.

We also thank Dr. Juan M. Taveras and Dr. Laurence L. Robbins for their encouragement. Both have used teaching methods similar to this one.

The cases we have used are based on material in the active file and the Radiology Teaching Collection at the Massachusetts General Hospital. We are grateful to the Williams & Wilkins Company of Baltimore, Maryland, for permission to use Figure 9, which originally appeared as Figure 542-A in *Radiologic Examination of the Colon* by Jack R. Dreyfuss, M.D., and Murray L. Janower, M.D., published in 1969. We are also grateful to Robert A. Grugan, M.D., of The Springfield Hospital Medical Center for his kind contribution of several films essential to the proper unfolding of one case.

Finally, we express our appreciation to Miss Selma I. Surman for her secretarial assistance, to Mr. Stanley Bennett for his photographic work, and to Mr. John Hanley of the W. B. Saunders Company, who was godfather to this volume and supplied the title.

L. F. S.

J. R. D.

C. S. L.

R. A. N.

CONTENTS

To use this volume properly, always begin with the historical vignette in section A. Decide on film findings, appropriate procedures and management before going on to each new section. Then thumb to the next section and specific page by referring to the notation in bold type on the right margin of each right hand page.

The division into sections has been done with the specific purpose of forcing the reader to pause before seeing the answers. If the system described above is used, the reader should be able to move from one section to another within five seconds.

PATIENT	PROBLEM	PART AND PAGE					
		A	B	C	D	E	F
Adumreb	Epigastric pain and vomiting	18	26	77	94	126	
Antonini	Blunt abdominal trauma	6	26	75	110		
Arachis	Cough and wheezing	3	25	52			
Bloat	Shortness of breath	15	30	82	111	124	134
Bloomer	Hypertension	7	44	69	91		
Cardoza	Urinary calculi	6	32	73	100		
Davenport	Fever of unknown origin	16	43	78	87	118	135
de Gautière	G.I. bleeding	17	30	76			
Eveready	Jaundice	5	47	56	88	122	
Feld	Recurrent abdominal pain and diarrhea	8	45	55	96	117	
Figtree	Hemoptysis	15	38	72	97		
Foon	Abdominal pain and distention	2	44	69	87		
Gaunt	Abdominal pain and bloody diarrhea	14	42				

PATIENT	PROBLEM	PART AND PAGE					
		A	B	C	D	E	F
Gave and Took	Motorcycle accident	9	31	73			
Grady	Head trauma	15	34				
Kent	Persistent cough	5	38	53	86	125	139
Lightfinger	Neck trauma	7	23	58	105		
Maladente	Swallowed foreign body	17	33				
Malatesta	Headache	3	23	74	101		
Mannerborn	Recurrent upper abdominal pain	12	34	70	106	128	
Pachooka	Child with diarrhea	11	38	79	99		
Parsons	Rejection by wife	13	27				
Pastone	Backache	17	25	77	95		
Reingold	Referred for abnormal chest film	19	24	79	109	116	134
Roach	Automobile accident	16	33	66	109	116	136
Rouge	Cough and hemoptysis	4	40	68	89	121	
Salem	Cough and fever	4	49	71	93		
Schock	Chest pain and shortness of breath	9	36	60	111	115	132
Sheldon	Right-sided abdominal pain	8	46	67	104	114	
Solent	Anorexia, weight loss, and vomiting	7	42	59	108		
Somers	Child with abdominal swelling	4	29	83	89	119	133
Stein	Left flank pain	12	38	62	103	118	137

PATIENT	PROBLEM	A	B	C	D	E	F
Stevens	Lymphoma	5	22	54	92	123	
Stone	Child with abdominal pain and constipation	3	24	61	107		
Tordu	Diarrhea, abdominal pain, and distention	17	41	83	94	120	
Vermilion	Bright red blood per rectum	16	48	57	90	114	
Walker	Dysphagia and ascites	11	33	80	102		
Waters	Hematuria	9	26	65	87	116	138
Watling	Vomiting	10	28	67	107		
Wilcox	Pedestrian struck by automobile	11	31	71	98	115	
Yglesias	Pathologic fracture	19	32	81			

PART A

PART A

Tai Foon, 68, ping pong instructor, is brought to the hospital by his family who say that he has been losing weight for several months and complaining of abdominal discomfort and constipation. On two occasions recently he passed a small amount of bright red blood with his stool. On the morning of admission he developed severe generalized abdominal pain and distention. Digital examination reveals an empty rectal ampulla. Except for a distended and tympanitic abdomen, the remainder of the physical examination is normal. Urine and stat blood studies are normal, and the patient is afebrile. You request a plain film of the abdomen (Fig. 1). What are your observations?

Continued Part B, page 44.

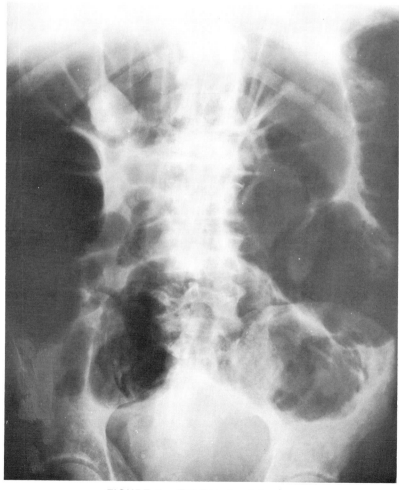

FIGURE 1. Tai Foon's abdomen

Rocco Malatesta, a 63 year old bus driver for the Golden Age Club, was well until a month ago when he developed a severe frontal headache. It did not respond to aspirin and in the past week has been constant.

You see him in clinic and discover that he has a blood pressure of 250/150. Funduscopic exam shows retinal hemorrhages. The remainder of his physical examination is unremarkable. He denies any previous history of hypertension, diabetes, or renal disease. Twenty years ago he had been hospitalized for a well-documented myocardial infarct.

The hemogram and electrolytes are normal. Urinalysis shows 2+ albumin with a sediment containing 5 RBCs and 2 WBCs per high-power field. How will you proceed with your work-up of this hypertensive patient?

Continued Part B, page 23.

Nicky Arachis, age 2, has been coughing all night. You see him in clinic. His mother says the coughing started yesterday afternoon following a quarrel during which he was knocked down by his older brother. He is afebrile and physical examination of his chest is normal. What will you do?

Continued Part B, page 25.

Penny Stone, a 5 year old girl, is brought to the hospital by her mother. She was well until last night when she began complaining of a generalized "tummy ache." Assuming that her daughter was constipated, Mrs. Stone administered an enema which produced some lumpy hard stool but did not provide any relief. The pain persisted through the night and is now localized to the right lower quadrant. This morning the child refused to eat breakfast. She denies nausea and vomiting; her mother states that she has been afebrile. There is no past history of urinary tract infection and the child has no dysuria or burning. Mrs. Stone adds that her daughter has complained of "tummy ache" several times during the past year.

On physical examination you observe a well-developed 5 year old girl who does not appear to be in distress. Her temperature is normal. Bowel sounds are present, although they are diminished. She points to the right lower quadrant of her abdomen, where you elicit tenderness to palpation without rebound tenderness. The remainder of the physical examination is normal; there is no rectal or costovertebral angle tenderness. What are you considering for a diagnosis and how will you proceed with your work-up?

Continued Part B, page 24.

Kevin Somers, a 2 year old child, was taken to his family doctor because of bilateral inguinal swelling. His mother was told that *Kevin* had hernias which might need an operation in the future. Now, 3 weeks later, *Kevin* has stopped eating, is listless, and has an enlarging abdomen. Mrs. Somers is worried and brings the child to see you in the Emergency Room.

You find a chronically ill child with diminished skin turgor, a clear chest, but an enlarged doughy abdomen and bilateral firm scrotal swellings. The bowel sounds are normal. The initial hemogram shows Hct 33, WBC 11,400 with 51 polys, 33 lymphocytes, and 10 monocytes. The urinalysis is normal, but the stool is guaiac-positive. How will you proceed?

Continued Part B, page 29.

Caleb P. Salem is a 56 year old shipwright who has smoked heavily for 30 years. He has a morning cough which is usually nonproductive, although occasionally he has seen flecks of blood in his sputum. He is now worried because he has twice coughed up frank blood and has a fever and right-sided chest pain. He has had no weight loss or night sweats.

Examining him, you hear a few wheezes over the right anterior chest, but no rales, egophony, or dullness. There is one shotty node in the right axilla. *Mr. Salem* is febrile with a temperature of 99.6° F., but the remainder of your exam is normal. The CBC and urinalysis are normal. Turn to *Part B, page 49,* for *Caleb's* chest film.

Lucy Rouge is the 59 year old cook (and frustrated poet) at the University Faculty Club. She is sent to you by the Board of Health because of an abnormal chest x-ray.

Mrs. Rouge tells you that she was well until 2 months ago when she developed a persistent cough with yellow sputum, but no blood. This cleared spontaneously, but recurred 2 weeks ago, and this time the sputum was bloody. She went to the Health Department where an x-ray was obtained and compared to those which she has had annually because of a positive TB skin test. The Health Department then referred her to you.

Lucy tells you that she has been smoking more than one pack of cigarettes daily since she was a girl. She is in good health and has no dyspnea, fatigue, or chest pain. Sometimes she sweats at night. She says she weighs 158 lbs, but you find that she weighs 141 lbs. Her vital signs are normal and except for a few wheezes in the left posterior chest, her physical examination and routine laboratory examination are completely normal. Her chest film is in *Part B, page 40.*

Alfred Stevens, a 22 year old graduate student, comes to the medical clinic for a checkup. He has been feeling tired since mid-term exams 3 months ago and has lost 8 lbs in the past month. Other than easy tiring, *Mr. Stevens* feels well. He has had no fever or chills and describes his general health as good. He drinks only socially and does not smoke.

Mr. Stevens is worried but does not appear ill. His vital signs are normal. You see no needle marks, bruises, rashes, or petechiae, and find no lymphadenopathy or splenomegaly. Cardiorespiratory and abdominal examinations are normal. There is no organomegaly. The initial CBC and urinalysis are normal. How will you evaluate this patient? What are your tentative diagnoses? Please turn to *Part B, page 22.*

Amanda Kent: You have completed your internship and are now a medical officer in the Air Force. *Amanda Kent,* a 40 year old Master Sergeant in the WAF sees you on sick call because of a persistent cough. She claims to be in good health and wants only a prescription for "G.I. gin" (elixir of terpin hydrate). She says the cough began with a cold 2 months ago and is productive of only scant amounts of clear sputum. She denies fevers, chills, chest pain, or weight loss.

Sergeant Kent looks well but has a temperature of 99.4° F., and, hearing sticky rales in the left posterior chest, you obtain a white count and differential, a sputum sample, and a chest x-ray. The results of these examinations are in *Part B, page 38.*

Jack Eveready, a 32 year old unemployed actor, comes to see you in medical clinic because he thinks he has jaundice. His general health has been good, but in the last 3 weeks he has felt tired and thinks his eyes are becoming yellow. His urine and stool have not changed in color, but he has lost his appetite for food and cigarettes and has experienced 2 attacks of right-sided abdominal pain. He has no fatty food intolerance. *Jack* eats raw shellfish, drinks heavily on the weekends, smokes pot, and has tried heroin, but claims not to use it habitually.

Mr. Eveready does have a slight yellowish cast to his sclerae, but is not grossly icteric. There are no needle marks or spiders. His liver is not palpable, but is tender to percussion. You cannot feel his spleen, and the rest of his physical examination is entirely normal. Admission CBC, urinalysis, and EKG are normal except for trace bile in the urine and a white count of 12,600 with a normal differential. How will you evaluate this patient? Please turn to *Part B, part 47.*

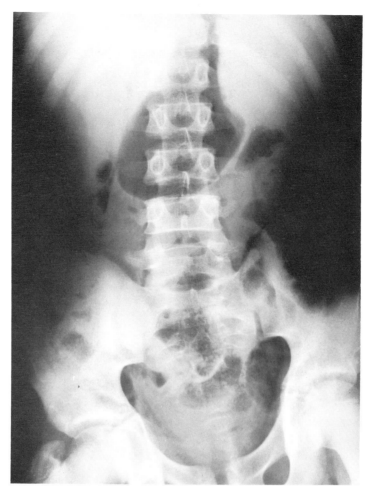

FIGURE 2. Vittorio Antonini's abdomen

Vittorio Antonini, age 12, was kicked in the stomach at football practice two days ago and has complained of stomach ache ever since. He is brought to the hospital by his mother. The pain has increased steadily and now he lies in bed, knees flexed, thrashing from side to side. You examine him and find what appears to be an enlarged tender spleen. His vital signs are stable. Figure 2 is his plain film.

Continued Part B, page 26.

Adalena Cardoza, age 35, is admitted from clinic to your service because of abdominal pain for 5 days. She tells you she has had several attacks of urinary tract infection and passed 4 stones in the past 12 years. She is febrile (T=100° F.) and stat urinalysis shows the presence of many WBCs and a few RBCs. What studies will you plan for her initially?

Continued Part B, page 32.

Henry Mountjoy Solent, age 71, retired Senior Captain and former Master of the transatlantic liner *Gigantic*, is referred to the hospital by a physician to whom he has complained of anorexia and weight loss. *Captain Solent* was in blooming good health until about 3 months ago when he first became aware of frequent gaseous distress without pain and the insidious onset of anorexia. In the past 2 months his weight has dropped from 190 to 170 lbs, and he has felt increasingly weak and has been still further discomforted by abdominal bloating. He has no pain but during the past 2 days he has been quite nauseated and on 4 occasions has vomited what little food he had eaten.

When you see the patient, he is extremely anxious and pale and appears dehydrated. He has had no previous serious illnesses or surgery and he has no other complaints. On examination you find only abdominal distention and what palpation suggests to be a large, fluid-filled structure in the abdomen. Studies show BP 128/80, T 99.0° F., P 64, weight 165 lbs., urinalysis normal, stool guaiac-negative, WBC 6900, and Hct 36.

What x-ray studies would you consider doing first?

Continued Part B, page 42.

Violet Bloomer, a 59 year old housewife, volunteered for an experimental computer analysis of her health profile. Her blood pressure and electrocardiogram were said to be abnormal. An intravenous pyelogram was subsequently noted to be abnormal but is now lost. *Mrs. Bloomer's* blood pressure is unstable on rauwolfia, and she is sent to you to see if she has a surgically treatable cause of hypertension.

You elicit the additional history that she has had intermittent urinary tract infections for 6 years, including one episode of fevers, chills, and right back pain which responded to treatment with sulfonamides. Turn to *Part B, page 44* for the admission chest film and intravenous pyelogram. What do you make of them?

Clyde Lightfinger: 17 year old *Clyde Lightfinger* is an injured accident victim. He was the driver of a stolen convertible that hit a truck after skidding on wet pavement five hours ago. Two detectives who had been pursuing the car accompany the young man to the emergency ward. *Lightfinger* says that he was briefly unconscious after the impact and awoke a few moments later with severe neck pain, sprawled across the passenger seat. His only neurologic complaint is numbness in the fourth and fifth fingers of each hand.

You observe an extremely anxious young man in acute painful distress. He walks supporting his head with his hands. He refuses to move his head or neck in any direction. What is your diagnosis? What will you do first?

Continued Part B, page 23.

Lorraine Sheldon, age 61, is brought to the hospital by ambulance shortly after she collapsed on stage at the Shubert Theatre while attempting to play Ophelia in *Hamlet*. When you first see her in the emergency room she is fully conscious and complains only of nausea and epigastric pain. She tells you that her gallbladder and appendix were removed 26 years ago and that part of her stomach was removed because of duodenal ulcer disease 3 years ago.

For the past several months she has had increasingly frequent episodes of right lower and upper abdominal pain, sometimes lasting up to 12 hours and often followed by diarrhea. This morning she felt nauseated and had moderately severe abdominal pain all day. She took only tea for lunch and supper and had several episodes of watery diarrhea during the afternoon, but with no relief of pain. There was no understudy to take over her role of Ophelia, so she went on in the tradition of the theatre. During the play, the pain increased in severity and became localized in the right upper abdomen. Just as Hamlet told her "Get thee to a nunnery," she fainted.

On physical examination *Miss Sheldon* looks several years younger than her stated age. Examination shows BP 130/80, T 98.4° F., P 80. The only positive findings are abdominal. There is a tender fullness palpable in the right upper quadrant and extending along the right side of the abdomen to the right lower quadrant. No spasm, guarding, or rebound tenderness. The bowel sounds are absent. Rectal examination is negative; a finger specimen of the stool is 2+ guaiac-positive. Stat blood studies: WBC 11,200, Hct 32. Urinalysis negative. What initial x-ray studies would you request?

Continued Part B, page 46.

Hannah Feld, age 23, arrives at the hospital with a temperature of 99.6°, complaining of diarrhea, nausea, and right lower quadrant pain. On questioning it develops that her complaints are actually of 2 weeks' duration and that this is her third similar episode in 5 months. She spent last summer in Israel working on a kibbutz and while there had her first attack of sharp, intermittent right lower quadrant pain and several loose bowel movements unassociated with meals or activity. She ran a low-grade fever. Her symptoms lasted 7 days and then gradually abated. A month after her return home, she had another attack of right lower quadrant pain, diarrhea, and evening temperature elevation. X-ray studies of the G.I. tract and colon were negative and blood studies were normal. She again improved after a week.

At present she appears pale and somewhat thin for her build. Blood studies show WBC 12,000, Hb 10.1, Hct 32. The serum albumin is decreased and the corrected sedimentation rate is 60. Urinalysis is negative. On physical examination, there is a 10 cm area of fullness in the right lower quadrant which is very tender to palpation. Rectal examination reveals a tender fullness in the right vault. Hyperextension of the right leg elicits deep right lower quadrant pain.

You suspect appendicitis. What x-ray films would you request?

Continued Part B, page 45.

Pat Gave and Mike Took, both age 24, are inseparable companions. They have been injured riding their motorcycle. *Pat* obviously has a compound fracture of his femur. *Mike* has no apparent fractures but severe lacerations of his foot and scalp. You observe that *Pat's* fractured leg is 3 inches shorter than his normal one and obtain a stat AP radiograph (Figure 3).

Continued Part B, page 31.

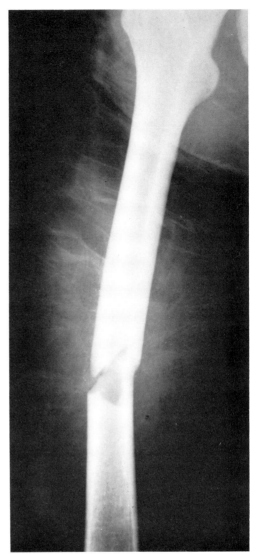

A–9

FIGURE 3. Pat's femur

Maximilian Schock, a 49 year old newspaper editor with a history of a previous myocardial infarction, was awakened by severe precordial chest pain associated with diaphoresis and shortness of breath. He was taken to an outside hospital where he was found to have distended neck veins, rales to the scapulae, and EKG evidence of a large anterior myocardial infarction. His admission chest film is in *Part B, page 36.* What do you make of it?

Ernest Waters is a 67 year old retired textile chemist who had always enjoyed good health until 2 months ago when he began noting increased urinary frequency associated with urgency. Several times each night he was awakened to void. In particular, he describes difficulty emptying his bladder, having to strain at the end of micturition. This morning he passed a small amount of blood with his urine. He denies burning or pain.

You observe an apprehensive, slender gentleman with a normal physical examination. Stat urinalysis confirms microscopic hematuria. The hemogram, BUN, and creatinine levels are all within normal limits. What are you considering as diagnostic possibilities and how will you proceed?

Continued Part B, page 26.

Carlton Watling, age 57, has been brought directly to the island hospital from his yacht, which has been anchored in St. George's Harbor for the past 2 days. Accompanying him is *Miss Cecily Mannerborn,* and it is immediately obvious that they have been partners in a floating bacchanal. Intermittently *Mr. Watling* vomits small quantities of liquid and food. He coughs frequently. *Cecily* mentions that her friend has been a patient at the hospital before and then quietly disappears into the night. No further history is obtainable.

You send for *Watling's* old medical record and then attempt a physical examination. The patient proves to be quite drunk and very combative. He denies any symptoms. His abdomen is distended but nontender. There are no peritoneal signs, but there is a succussion splash. His lungs seem clear but because of his constant chattering, it is difficult to be sure. Studies show BP 170/94, T 99.0° F., P 88, WBC 9000, stool specimen guaiac-negative.

His medical record arrives and you note that he has had 5 previous admissions. Three of them (18, 10, and 4 years ago) were for duodenal ulcer disease. In the past 7 years, he has also been admitted twice for acute alcoholism. You next pass a nasogastric tube and aspirate, with difficulty, nearly a liter of gastric contents (guaiac-negative). Then, because you fear he may have aspirated, you send him to x-ray for films of his chest (Figs. 4 and 5). Any clue to what is going on?

Continued Part B, page 28.

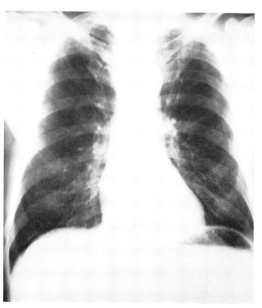

FIG. 4   FIG. 5

FIGURES 4 & 5. Carlton Watling's chest films

Mr. Johnny Walker, a 62 year old semi-retired ragtime piano player, comes to your clinic complaining of ankle swelling and increasing abdominal girth during the past 2 weeks. He was in good health until 6 months ago when he lost his appetite for food and alcohol. *Mr. Walker* was in the habit of "downing" several shots of whiskey each night when he was playing regularly at the Purple Garter Lounge.

Recently he began noting difficulty swallowing solid foods and placed himself on a soft diet. He believes he has lost over 40 lbs. There is no history of pain, jaundice, nausea, vomiting, or change in bowel habits. Although he admits to dyspnea on exertion, he denies angina, previous myocardial infarction, orthopnea, or paroxysmal nocturnal dyspnea.

You observe a thin, cachectic man with a markedly distended abdomen and peripheral edema. His conjunctiva are pale, but there is no scleral icterus. Dullness to percussion and diminished breath sounds are noted at the left base. Gross ascites is detected in the abdomen. His stool is 4+ guaiac-positive. The remainder of the physical examination is unremarkable. How will you proceed with this patient?

Continued Part B, page 33.

Chester Winston Wilcox, a 37 year old architect, was struck by a taxicab while chasing his springer spaniel across Park Avenue. An ambulance brought him directly to your emergency ward. *Mr. Wilcox* recalls that he was hit from the side, at the level of his hips, and was then "thrown" away from the car against the curb. He complains of excruciating pain about his pelvis as well as left flank pain.

You observe a well-developed man in acute painful distress with abrasions over his hands, arms, knees, and right hip. He is lying supine, hesitant to move. His vital signs are stable. Bowel sounds are present and the abdomen is soft; however, he has diffuse, variable abdominal tenderness. The pubic symphysis is extremely tender. He complains of abdominal pain on pubic compression. How will you manage this patient?

Continued Part B, page 31.

Tussy Pachooka, age 2, is brought to the hospital at 1:00 A.M. The worried young parents tell you she has had diarrhea all day, her stools being at first semi-formed, then liquid, and finally nothing but bloody mucus. She is screaming and has done so at intervals for 6 hours. She has not vomited. The past history is of no apparent relevance. Peristalsis is hyperactive. Palpation reveals a slight fullness on the right side of the abdomen but no rigidity. The abdomen is soft and neither distended nor tympanitic. What are the diagnostic possibilities? Has radiology anything to offer this patient that would help narrow the differential?

Continued Part B, page 38.

Cecily Mannerborn, age 37, consults you, stating that one week ago, while having tea on a friend's yacht anchored in St. George's Harbor, she experienced the rather sudden onset of left upper abdominal pain. It continued all afternoon, and on coming ashore that evening it seemed to intensify. She became quite nauseated and vomited several times. (She thought this was probably due to the fact that she had consumed too many sweets while on the yacht.) The next morning, the pain was somewhat better but she had a temperature of 100° F. She stayed in bed for several days. During the past 24 hours, the pain has recurred with the same intensity as on the first day while having tea afloat, and she is again nauseated and vomiting.

On further questioning, *Miss Mannerborn* reluctantly admits that she is an alcoholic and has been drinking heavily for a week. She further states that over the past 18 months she has had at least 4 similar episodes of abdominal pain and nausea, though in each case the pain was more midline, radiated through to the back, and was more severe than at present. She says that at another hospital she was told her attacks had been due to pancreatitis and that she also had mild diabetes. She has lost 21 lbs. in the past year.

On physical examination, the chest is dull to percussion with diminished breath sounds at the left base. There is moderate tenderness to deep palpation in the left upper quadrant of the abdomen. No mass is felt, however. Studies show BP 120/75, P 120, T 101° F., WBC 10,500, amylase 80, Hct 36, urinalysis 1+ glucose. What x-ray studies would you request?

Continued Part B, page 34.

Dr. Luke Stein, a 52 year old oceanography professor, was delivering his annual lecture on plankton migration in the Indian Ocean when he experienced the sudden onset of severe left flank pain. His concerned secretary, Kitty Karp, brought him directly to your emergency ward. He describes the pain as "excruciating, the worst pain I have ever felt." It occurs in spasms and radiates to the scrotum. He feels nauseated but has not vomited.

There is no past history of urinary tract symptoms or disease. He is known to your medical center for unexplained splenomegaly which was first detected 20 years ago following an expedition to Madagascar. No cause for his splenomegaly was ever determined. Three years ago he suffered from a herniated lumbar disc for which he underwent surgery in London. Since that time he has been in excellent health.

You observe an unusually distressed gentleman who is writhing on the examining table. No position provides relief. You elicit marked left flank and left costovertebral angle tenderness. There is spasm of the left rectus muscles. The spleen tip is palpable but not tender. His vital signs and the remainder of his physical examination are within normal limits. Which studies would you ask for first and what do you think they will show?

Continued Part B, page 38.

James Parsons, 61, machinist, is brought to the accident ward by neighbors after his wife hit him in the forehead with a shovel and shut the front door on his toes. He was returning home from prison after serving a 12 year term for armed robbery. His wife insists he is not her husband and that she never saw him before in her life.

As you examine him you note that he is a large, stooped, sad looking man with craggy features. He has no complaints other than the acute injuries, except for the fact that he has had to give up machine tooling because of bad eyesight that developed in prison. The bridge of his nose and lower forehead are very swollen and blue, and his foot is severely injured anteriorly with contusions about the toes. Figures 6 and 7 are films of his foot. Figure 8 is a later skull film (? fractured nose).

Continued Part B, page 27.

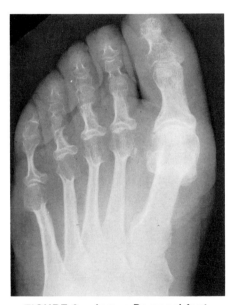

FIGURE 6. James Parsons' foot

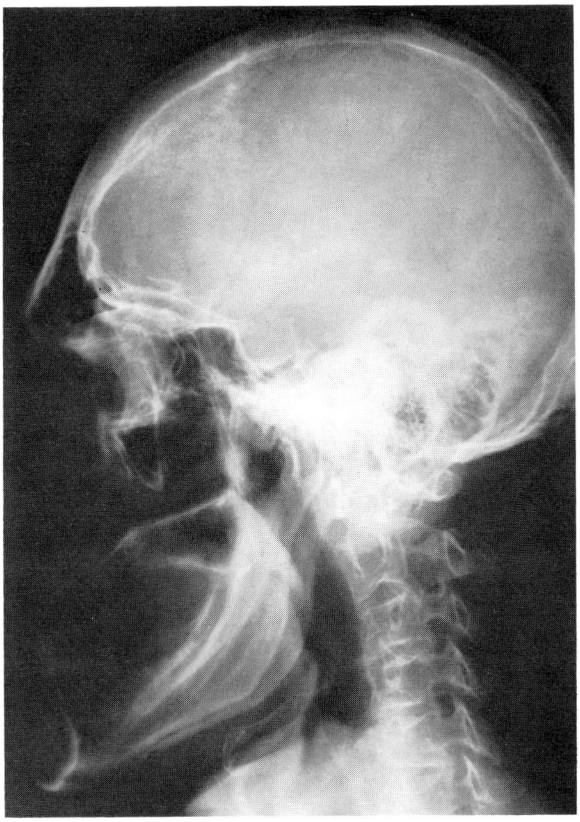

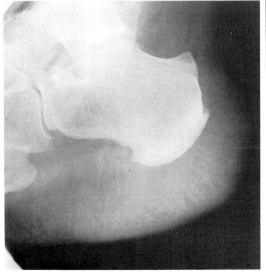

FIGURE 7. James Parsons' heel

FIGURE 8. James Parsons' skull

John Gaunt, 28, has been in the hospital for 10 days under treatment for ulcerative colitis. His disease was first diagnosed when he was a senior in college. Except for occasional exacerbations characterized by periods of abdominal cramps, diarrhea, and rectal bleeding, he has done well on low maintenance dosage of Azulfidine. Now hospitalized because of a recent flareup, he was responding to prednisone and increased Azulfidine therapy until 2 days ago.

Since then his condition has deteriorated, with alarming increase in abdominal pain, cramps, and bloody diarrhea. This morning his temperature has climbed to 105°F. and there has been a massive outpouring of blood from the rectum. On physical examination, his abdomen is hugely distended, exquisitely tender, and silent to auscultation. He rapidly goes into shock and you request a film of the abdomen to be followed by an emergency barium enema to see what has gone wrong. Here is the plain film of the abdomen (Fig. 9).

Continued Part B, page 42.

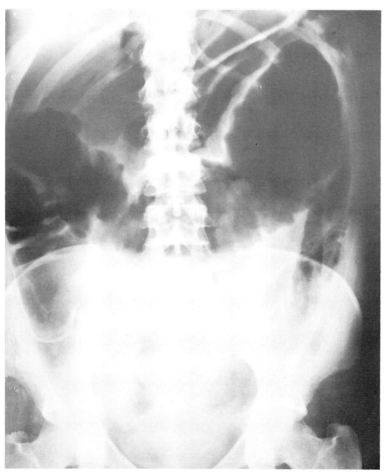

FIGURE 9. Plain film of John Gaunt's abdomen

Corey Bloat, a 46 year old short order cook, is brought by his brother to the emergency room because of shortness of breath. *Mr. Bloat* has enjoyed good health most of his adult life but in the past several years he has experienced occasional palpitations and intermittent ankle swelling. He does not have a history of heart disease and dates his present symptoms from a bout of the "flu" 3 weeks ago. His shortness of breath and an associated dull aching chest pain are both relieved if he remains sitting up.

Corey is visibly short of breath. His pulse is 130 and irregularly irregular, with a blood pressure of 140/80. His ankles are swollen and his neck veins distended at 45 degrees. Listening to his chest, you hear rales at the lung bases and soft irregular heart sounds. His EKG, CBC, and urinalysis are normal.

Please turn to *Part B, page 30,* for *Mr. Bloat's* admission chest film. Then decide how you will proceed.

Ms. Phoenicia Figtree, 52 year old veteran reporter for the *Metropolitan Gazette,* recently noticed an increase in her usual "smoker's cough." She has been smoking 2 packages of unfiltered cigarettes a day for over 30 years. Two weeks ago her regular morning cough began to persist throughout the day. She also noticed the onset of a wheeze and shortness of breath on exertion. Tonight she coughed up a small amount of bright red blood and took a taxi cab directly to your emergency ward.

During the physical examination, you observe an anxious, thin female with an audible wheeze. She shows you a piece of Kleenex stained with red blood. On chest auscultation you localize the wheeze to the left side. There are bronchial breath sounds on the left as well. The remainder of the examination is normal. She is afebrile. Which study will you request? What do you think it will show?

Continued Part B, page 38.

Theophilus Grady, 36, is brought roaring drunk into the accident ward by his similarly afflicted companions after an altercation in a bar during which he was knocked down, hitting his head on the edge of a table. He is bleeding from the right ear and has an ecchymosis over the right mastoid. He has no gross neurologic deficits; however, a complete neurologic examination cannot be performed on this inebriated patient. His "friends" want to take him home. What should you do?

Continued Part B, page 34.

Dollface Davenport, a 64 year old retired mobster, comes to clinic complaining of daily fevers and chills which began 7 weeks ago. A local doctor diagnosed the flu and prescribed tetracycline, but his fevers have continued and *Dollface* is worried. He is not eating and has lost 22 lbs. in the past 2 months.

You take a careful history and are able to elicit no further symptoms except occasional low back pain. There are no cardiorespiratory symptoms, no changes in bowel or urinary habits, no rashes, and no exposures or inoculations.

Mr. Davenport is a thin, anxious man with a rectal temperature of 100.4°F. Physical examination reveals a soft systolic murmur in the third left interspace and a liver which is palpable but not tender and not enlarged. The rest of his examination, including a rectal exam, is normal. Laboratory work immediately available includes a white count of 10,400 with 8 bands and no eosinophils. There are 4 to 8 WBCs per high-power field on urinalysis. How will you proceed? Please turn to *Part B, page 43.*

Colette Vermilion, 57, President of Les Amours de Cheri Perfume Co., is seeing you for her annual executive checkup and mentions that she has had some rectal bleeding for the past 2 months and it has been bright red. She denies any other G.I. tract symptoms.

Physical examination including rectal examination is negative—no hemorrhoids. Stat hematocrit is normal. You next perform sigmoidoscopy and see nothing but a few drops of blood coming from above the reach of the scope. What do you do next?

Continued Part B, page 48.

Jay Roach, a "hip" 26 year old graduate student, was involved in an automobile accident 1 hour ago. While driving home from a late party he lost control of his small convertible on a sharp turn and struck a light pole. An ambulance transported him to your emergency ward. You find a long-haired, slightly confused young man, lying on a stretcher in acute painful distress.

Mr. Roach does not recall the details of the accident well. He last remembers hitting his left knee against the dashboard and then "blacking out." He complains of severe left hip pain and warns you not to move his left leg. He also describes right lower chest pain.

His vital signs are stable. There are abrasions over his forehead, right chest wall, left hand, and left knee. The lungs are clear. Bowel sounds are normal and the abdomen is soft and nontender. The left hip is flexed and adducted but not rotated. The remainder of the examination is unremarkable.

Although he answers questions slowly and somewhat inappropriately, he is well oriented without any neurologic deficit. He denies drinking at the party and there is no odor of alcohol on his breath. You notice a package of strawberry flavored cigarette paper in his left shirt pocket. How will you manage this patient?

Continued Part B, page 33.

Ninette de Gautière, 20, college student, is brought to the emergency ward of your hospital after she fainted in class this morning. She tells you she has been in no pain of any kind but did pass a large black stool yesterday. She is in apparently excellent general health except for some pallor and understandable anxiety. Vital signs are normal but the hematocrit is 34. What should you do first?

Continued Part B, page 30.

Pierre Claude Tordu, 56, the noted Chef de Cuisine from Juan-les-Pins, is forced to interrupt his lecture tour and enter the hospital. He tells you he has been suffering from diarrhea for the past week, 3 to 4 semisolid stools a day with a great deal of mucus but no blood. He consulted a doctor in another city who believed *Monsieur Tordu's* symptoms were due to a strenuous tour schedule and the change from his usual diet. Yesterday the patient began to have crampy lower abdominal pain. He gave himself an enema, which was productive of a small amount of fecal material but no gas. The pain steadily increased in severity, his abdomen became distended and tense, and he consulted another physician who recommended admission to the hospital.

On physical examination, there is moderate abdominal tenderness and you can palpate dilated bowel in the left upper and lower quadrants. High-pitched tinkles are heard in the abdomen on auscultation. T 99.4° F., BP 145/80, P 90, WBC 7,300.

What x-ray examination would you request?

Continued Part B, page 41.

A–17

Mrs. Donna Maladente, a 26 year old young mother, arrives at your office with a letter from her dentist. It states that she has just swallowed a gold cap intended for a molar. He suggests that you "order an x-ray plate of her abdomen." She is anxious but completely asymptomatic. Do you arrange for the "plate"?

Continued Part B, page 33.

Mary Pastone, 72, complains of pain in her lower back increasing gradually over 2 years. She keeps house for her widowed son and his 2 children. She can recall no particular trauma to her back but is certain it always hurts more on Fridays when she carries in bags of groceries for the weekend. What film studies are in order?

Continued Part B, page 25.

Dr. Notlimah Adumreb, 33, has just returned from a month's vacation in his native land. While there, he was twice distressed by a dull aching in his right upper quadrant and epigastrium. He also felt slight nausea. Each time he obtained relief by placing himself on small bland meals for several days and taking frequent gulps of a liquid antacid. During the flight back to this country, he ate a rather large lunch, and 2 hours later his symptoms returned with a vengeance. The dull aching rapidly progressed to severe epigastric pain and he became nauseated. Just before the plane landed, he was forced to go to the lavatory and vomit. There was no gross blood in the vomitus. He took a taxi directly from the airport to the emergency ward of your hospital.

On physical examination there is a sense of fullness in the epigastric and right upper quadrant areas. No definite mass is defined and there is no tenderness. T 98.8°F., P 90, WBC 10,500, Hct 42. Urinalysis is negative except for 1 RBC and 1 to 3 WBCs per high-power field. He vomits once more (guaiac-negative) and feels somewhat better. You persuade him to remain overnight and he is given nothing to eat. The next morning further laboratory reports reveal normal liver function studies and normal electrolytes. The amylase is 12. He is then sent to the x-ray department for an upper gastrointestinal series. Here are 2 of the films from that study (Figs. 10 and 11).

Continued Part B, page 26.

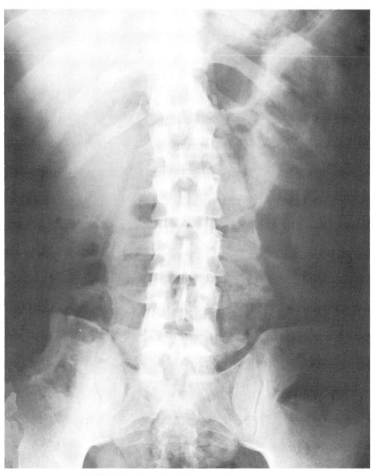

FIGURE 10. Dr. Adumreb's plain film

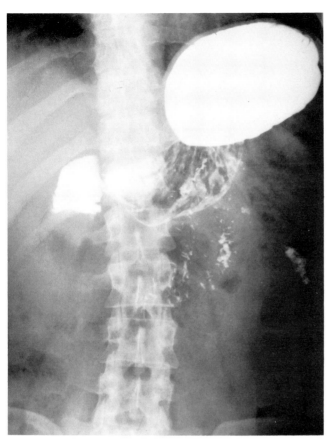

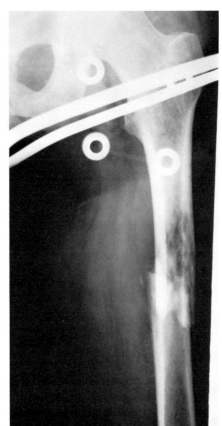

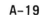

A-19

FIGURE 11. Representative film from Adumreb's upper gastrointestinal series

FIGURE 12. Roberto's femur

Roberto Yglesias, 71, is admitted by ambulance in great pain after a fall on the highly polished floor of his local dance studio. His left thigh is painful and swollen, but his vital signs are stable, and he appears to be in excellent health. Figure 12 is the stat AP film of his femur obtained in the accident room.

Continued Part B, page 32.

Ruby Hobson Reingold IV, the 53 year old wife of a Park Avenue physician, is referred to you by her family doctor because of an abnormal chest film. He had obtained the chest film to evaluate a 4 day history of myalgias, cough, and pleuritic right chest pain. *Mrs. Reingold* is now entirely asymptomatic.

At the time of your examination, no further pertinent history can be obtained. The patient feels herself to be in good health. She has never smoked. Her last chest x-ray, 4 years ago, was reportedly normal. Physical examination reveals a healthy, well-nourished, middle-aged woman with normal vital signs. There are no breast masses and the remainder of the examination including a pelvic exam is normal. The CBC is normal. Urinalysis reveals 2 to 4 RBCs per high-power field. Please turn to *Part B, page 24,* for her chest film.

Clyde Lightfinger: *(Continued from page 7)* Immediately you immobilize his neck with a plastic collar to prevent possible spinal cord injury from a suspected cervical spine fracture. You then examine him for any neurologic deficits and find none. With the exception of the neck, his initial physical examination is unremarkable. After warning the radiologist and technician of a possible cervical spine fracture, you send the patient to the radiology department. With the plastic collar in place, survey AP and cross-table lateral films of the cervical spine can be obtained in the supine position. No movement or physical effort is required of the patient. The odontoid may be well visualized in the AP projection by centering the x-ray beam through the patient's opened mouth. The films are reproduced in *Part C, page 58.* What is your opinion of them?

B–23

Rocco Malatesta: *(Continued from page 3)* Your work-up will entail a search for both renal and nonrenal causes of *Mr. Malatesta's* hypertension. You request a *hypertensive* intravenous urogram.

This study differs from the standard IVU by including films taken at 1, 2, 3, 4, and 5 minutes. In the normal patient the nephrogram, or parenchymal phase, is best seen on the 1 minute film. It is produced by contrast substance in the nephrons. Contrast should be seen in the calyces on the 3 or 4 minute film. Delay in visualization of the nephrogram or of the calyces reflects disease of the renal arteries or renal parenchyma which may be responsible for a patient's hypertension.

Mr. Malatesta should have a urine culture, and blood samples should be drawn to rule out possible diabetic nephrosclerosis.

You will begin your investigation of nonrenal causes of hypertension by ordering a plasma cortisol level as an evaluation of adrenal cortex activity. Also you request a 24 hour urine collection to measure vanillylmandelic acid (VMA) excretion rate in order to rule out pheochromocytoma.

Did you request a chest film? Please turn to *Part C, page 74* to interpret the hypertensive IVU.

Penny Stone: *(Continued from page 3)* The clinical picture certainly suggests acute appendicitis, although several classic manifestations are absent. Her chief complaint of pain, now persistent and localized, as well as the evidence for constipation ("hard, lumpy stools") favors the diagnosis of appendicitis. However, there has been no history of nausea, vomiting, or fever. She has right lower quadrant tenderness, but no rebound or rectal tenderness. In your differential, you are probably also including urinary tract infection and mesenteric adenitis.

You order a stat urinalysis and hemogram. After the samples are taken, you send the patient for supine and upright films of the abdomen and chest films (she is a surgery candidate). Consider what these films may show and then turn to *Part C, page 61.*

Ruby Hobson Reingold IV: *(Continued from page 19)* Here are *Mrs. Reingold's* abnormal chest films (Figs. 15 and 16). What do you see?

There is a sharply defined, more or less spherical lesion near the right cardiophrenic angle. Reasonable diagnostic possibilities must include tumor or inflammatory masses in the lung. Hamartoma, primary or metastatic carcinoma, or tuberculoma could appear like this. Have you considered any other diagnoses? What further data or procedures do you need? Turn to *Part C, page 79.*

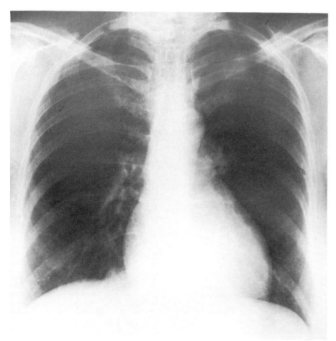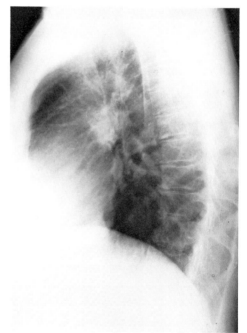

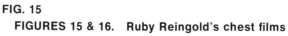

FIG. 15 **FIG. 16**
FIGURES 15 & 16. Ruby Reingold's chest films

Nicky Arachis: *(Continued from page 3)* If you asked for a "PA chest film stat reading," you probably got a telephoned report, "Negative chest," on Figure 17. Will you let the child go home?

Continued Part C, page 52.

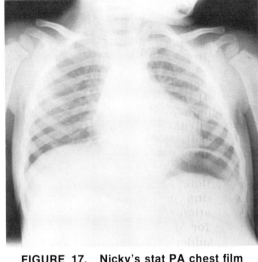

FIGURE 17. Nicky's stat PA chest film

Mary Pastone: *(Continued from page 17)* Films of her lumbar spine and pelvis are certainly indicated and here they are (Figs. 18 and 19). Do they suggest a diagnosis? What will you do next?

Continued Part C, page 77.

B-25

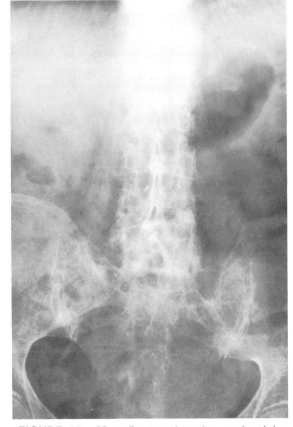

FIGURE 18. Mary Pastone's spine and pelvis

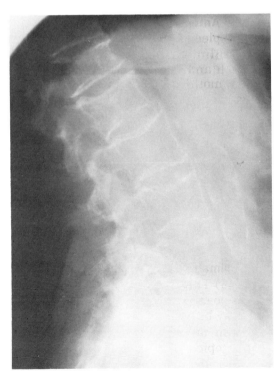

FIGURE 19. Mary Pastone's spine

Ernest Waters: *(Continued from page 9)* Of course you would request an intravenous urogram. His symptoms suggest bladder outlet obstruction, most frequently caused by benign prostatic hypertrophy. If this is the case, you will want to evaluate his upper urinary tracts to rule out hydronephrotic changes secondary to obstruction. In addition, you want to search for evidence of infection which so frequently accompanies urinary tract obstruction.

Having performed a normal rectal examination, you also consider other causes for *Mr. Waters'* symptoms. Both large bladder tumors and bladder stones may present as bladder outlet obstruction. Gross hematuria is a common symptom for both of these entities, especially when accompanied by cystitis. It should be kept in mind, however, that episodes of gross hematuria may occur with uncomplicated benign prostatic hypertrophy; dilated veins which develop at the bladder neck may rupture when the patient strains to void.

When reviewing *Mr. Waters'* urogram you should also be alert for signs of renal and ureteral neoplasms, calculi, renal cysts, and tuberculous infections. These conditions may produce hematuria. Did you ask for a chest film? Please turn to *Part C, page 65* and evaluate the films provided.

Vittorio Antonini: *(Continued from page 6)* The spleen is definitely enlarged on the plain film, indenting the air-filled stomach and displacing it medially. You tell his mother that the spleen is enlarged and then she tells you that she has thalassemia and that the boy's spleen was felt once before during a febrile illness several years ago. What will you do now?

Continued Part C, page 75.

Dr. Notlimah Adumreb: *(Continued from page 18)* The plain film of the abdomen shows no striking findings. The right kidney may be slightly larger than the left. The film taken after completion of the fluoroscopic study confirms that the stomach and duodenal cap are normal, but there is near complete obstruction of the second portion of the duodenum. The barium ends in a horizontal cut-off suggesting the presence of extrinsic pressure rather than an intrinsic lesion. The right kidney still appears slightly larger than might be expected.

Dr. Adumreb is again persuaded to remain in the hospital and is treated with IV fluids, intermittent gastric suction, and mild sedation for his restlessness and minimal complaints of right upper abdominal distress. What studies would you consider requesting next?

Continued Part C, page 77.

James Parsons: *(Continued from page 13)* The nasal bones are almost always "burned out" in lateral skull films. If you suspect nasal fracture, you should ask for films of the nasal bones. A lateral film with a very light exposure and a "bite-wing" view will be obtained for you. This is done with a special small film held between the teeth and a vertical x-ray beam. Nasal fractures are very difficult to diagnose without such studies.

(Figures 20 and 21, another patient, show a nasal fracture.)

Mr. Parsons has no fractures, but he *does* have an enlarged, ballooned-out sella and an excessively long mandible, indicating acromegaly. This diagnosis is also suggested by the extraordinary thickness of the soft tissues underneath the calcaneus. The heel pad normally measures no more than 25 mm. On the original film this heel pad measured 30 mm.

Soft tissue thickening and renewed cartilage and bone growth also account for the characteristic hand film with gross distal tufts, wide soft tissues, and widened joint spaces with thick cartilage (Fig. 22). Even an acromegalic can present with acute trauma, and now we know why his wife did not recognize him and what kind of visual fields he has.

End of Case

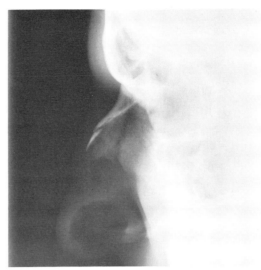

FIG. 20

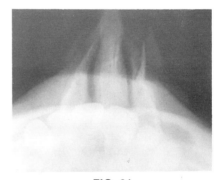

FIG. 21
FIGURES 20 & 21.   A broken nose

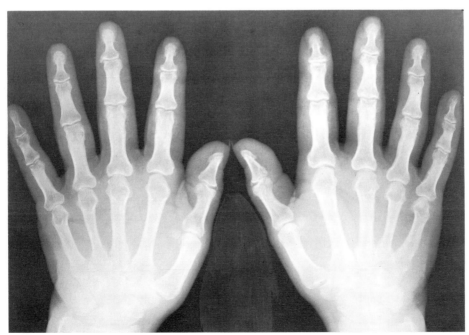

FIGURE 22.   James Parsons' hands

Carlton Watling: *(Continued from page 10)* His lungs are clear without evidence of aspiration pneumonitis. The nasogastric tube passes down the esophagus and into the stomach. The significant observation on these chest films: although you have already withdrawn nearly a liter of fluid from *Mr. Watling's* stomach, there still is a very formidable gastric fluid level. You next obtain an upright film of the abdomen (Fig. 23).

The impressive gastric fluid level, the wide curving sweep of the gastric tube, and the general background "grayness" of the left side of the abdomen all suggest that there is still a tremendous amount of fluid in the stomach, perhaps as much as another 5 liters. (The round, metallic-like objects at the bottom of the film are snaps on the patient's boxer shorts.) What do you do?

Continued Part C, page 67.

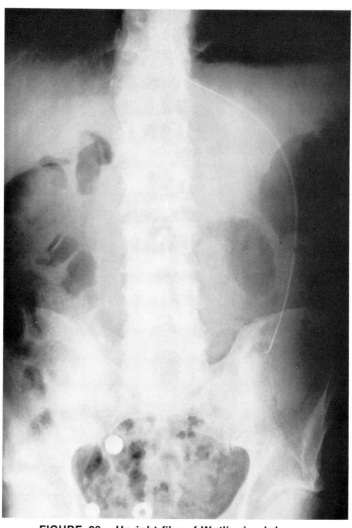

FIGURE 23. Upright film of Watling's abdomen

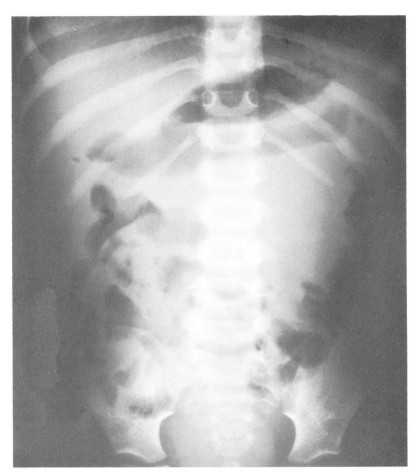

FIGURE 24. Kevin's abdomen

Kevin Somers: *(Continued from page 4)* You admit *Kevin* to the hospital. Here is a supine film of his abdomen. How would you interpret it?

There is no bowel gas in the left mid-abdomen. However, the bowel you can see is normal in caliber, and it is possible to trace gas all the way through the intestine. That is the body of the stomach at the top of the film. The edges of the abdomen are framed by what is probably colon, fixed by its short mesentery. The sigmoid, with a longer mesentery, may be lifted out of the pelvis by the bladder or

it may be empty of gas. The irregular collections of gas to the right of the spine are probably in small bowel. Therefore, the abdominal swelling is not due to obstruction of bowel by an incarcerated hernia which should have been one of your preliminary diagnoses. Nor is this ascites; if it were, the gas-filled bowel would float centrally in a supine patient.

What then are you feeling in *Kevin's* abdomen? Physical examination reveals a lumpy abdomen but no large mass. How will you proceed?

Please turn to *Part C, page 83.*

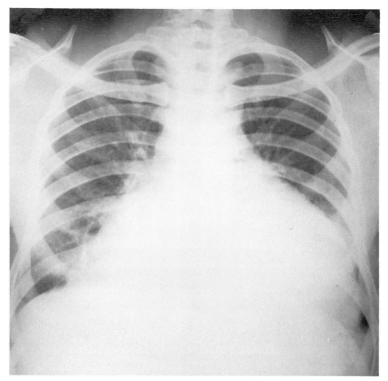

FIGURE 25.   Corey Bloat's admission chest film

Corey Bloat: *(Continued from page 15)* The admission chest film (Fig. 25) shows gross, symmetrical cardiac enlargement. The pulmonary vasculature is only slightly distended. There are no pleural effusions or infiltrates, and *Mr. Bloat* is not in florid pulmonary edema. What are your tentative diagnoses? How are you going to evaluate this heart?

Please turn to *Part C, page 82.*

Ninette de Gautière: *(Continued from page 17)* Type and cross-match her blood, of course. Barium studies can wait. Admit her, put in a CVP line, and request stat laboratory studies appropriate to an acute G.I. bleeder. The most likely diagnosis in this patient is duodenal ulcer.

Painless hemorrhage in young people with unsuspected peptic ulcer disease is not at all rare. Determining the source of bleeding by any sort of x-ray study is of secondary importance compared with supportive therapy. You insert a nasogastric tube. The gastric aspirate is guaiac-negative.

If the hematocrit drops or is very hard to stabilize, you may then decide to send this patient to the floor via radiology for an *emergency* barium study. How will you make out the requisition if you decide to do this?

Continued Part C, page 76.

Pat and Mike: *(Continued from page 9)* Figure 26 is a film made with *Pat's* leg in traction. A fourth year medical student comments that "it looks as if something is missing." (Figure 27 is *Mike's* foot film.)

Continued Part C, page 73.

Chester Winston Wilcox: *(Continued from page 11)* Mr. *Wilcox* has suffered pelvic and abdominal trauma; blood loss and shock are potential hazards for this patient. Initially you draw blood samples for blood typing and cross-matching in the event that a transfusion may be required. You also send a sample for stat hematocrit. A central venous pressure line is inserted to evaluate the patient's fluid requirements, and a Foley catheter is installed to monitor urine output. No gross hematuria is observed. You request frequent checking of vital signs.

Mr. *Wilcox* clinically appears to have a fractured pelvis. The etiology of the left flank pain is unclear, but you are concerned about possible renal trauma. He is taken to the radiology department for AP chest, abdomen, and pelvis films as his initial radiographic studies.

Please turn to *Part C, page 71,* to interpret these films.

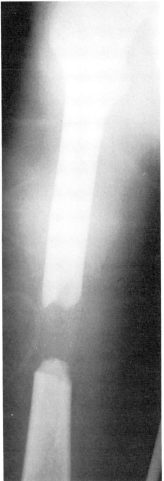

B–31

FIGURE 26. Pat's leg in traction

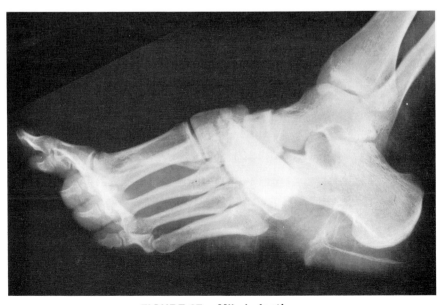

FIGURE 27. Mike's foot!

Roberto Yglesias: *(Continued from page 19)* This is not a straightforward fracture. The midshaft of the femur is riddled with irregular areas of bone destruction. A diagnosis of pathologic fracture is inescapable. What sort of tumor might this be? How will you proceed?

Continued Part C, page 81.

Adalena Cardoza: *(Continued from page 6)* You will certainly have requested a plain film of her abdomen and probably an intravenous urogram to follow. (Did you remember that a plain film, checked by the radiologist before proceeding, is an automatic first step for an excretory study and therefore not necessary to request separately?) Figure 28 is part of a delayed film from *Miss Cardoza's* urogram. How would you interpret it?

Continued Part C, page 73.

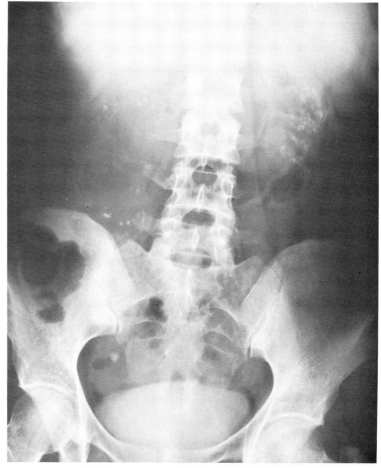

FIGURE 28. Film from Adalena's IVU

Johnny Walker: (*Continued from page 11*) Without other manifestations of cardiac disease, *Mr. Walker's* ascites and peripheral edema can be assumed to be secondary to liver failure. Although he admits to ethanolism, and cirrhosis is a consideration, his history of anorexia, significant weight loss, and dysphagia suggests malignant disease.

Stat hemogram reveals a hypochromic, microcytic anemia with a hematocrit of 21 per cent. This finding accounts for his exertional dyspnea and is consistent with blood loss from the gastrointestinal tract in a patient with guaiac-positive stools. Liver function studies confirm the expected hypoalbuminemia with diminished total protein. The urinalysis is normal.

Please turn to *Part C, page 80,* and review the initial radiographic studies which you have reqested: PA and lateral chest films and a plain abdominal film.

Donna Maladente: (*Continued from page 17*) In a young married woman you should take a menstrual history before requesting any type of abdominal x-ray examination. On questioning *Mrs. Maladente*, you learn that she has in fact missed her last 2 periods and knows that she is pregnant. Only when absolutely necessary should one expose a pregnant patient to radiation in the first trimester.

B-33

This patient will most likely pass the gold cap without incident. You advise the patient to examine her stools for the foreign body and to return only in the unlikely event that gastrointestinal symptoms develop.

As for requesting "plates," glass plates haven't been used since long before your time.

End of Case

Jay Roach: (*Continued from page 16*) After drawing blood for stat hematocrit and for type and cross-matching, you insert a central venous pressure line. His urine is clear and a sample is sent for analysis.

You send *Mr. Roach* to the radiology department for survey AP views of the chest, abdomen, and pelvis (which will include the left hip). You also request AP and cross-table lateral views of the skull because of his history of unconsciousness and forehead abrasions.

Please turn to *Part C, page 66* and interpret the films reproduced there.

Theophilus Grady: (*Continued from page 15*) You do not need to demonstrate a basilar skull fracture now; you have strong evidence that *Mr. Grady* has one (Battle's sign is present). The demonstration of basilar skull fractures requires special positioning and cooperation which will not be obtained from this patient at this time. You should arrange for "survey AP, lateral, and Towne's projection films of the skull" to rule out any other fractures that are not clinically apparent. You are especially interested in ruling out a depressed fracture or a fracture crossing a middle meningeal artery groove. You admit him for observation and begin antibiotics. You can search for the basilar fracture later when he is better able to cooperate.

End of Case

Cecily Mannerborn: (*Continued from page 12*) Because of the physical findings, films of the abdomen and chest are obtained (Figs. 29, 30, and 31). After looking them over, what do you see that is abnormal?

Continued Part C, page 70.

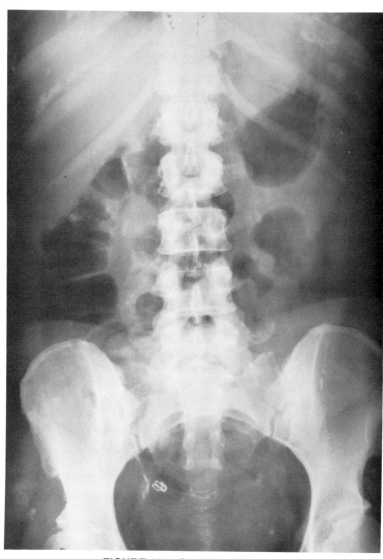

FIGURE 29. Cecily's abdomen

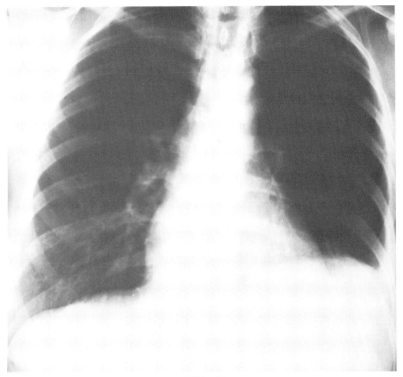

FIG. 30

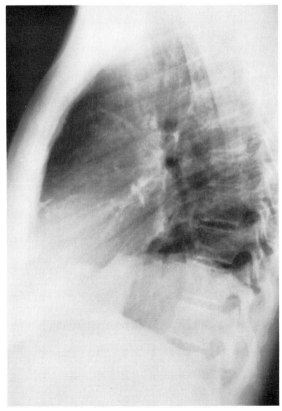

FIG. 31
FIGURES 30 & 31. Cecily's chest

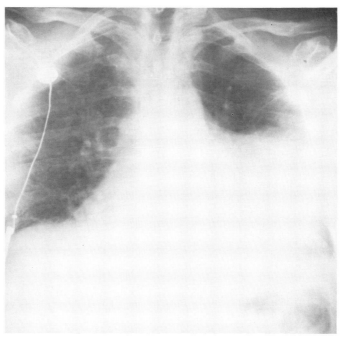

FIGURE 32. Maximilian Schock's emergency chest film

Maximilian Schock: *(Continued from page 9)* This portable AP film (Fig. 32) was obtained without moving *Mr. Schock* from his bed. (You can see the cardiac monitor leads overlying the chest.) Even though this is a portable film, it is unquestionably abnormal with a large mass arising from or adjacent to the left ventricle. With the history of a previous myocardial infarction, this was interpreted as a large left ventricular aneurysm. The EKG indicates a new infarction. *Mr. Schock* was treated conservatively and did well. PA and lateral chest films (Figs. 33 and 34) were obtained prior to discharge. These films confirm the size and shape of the aneurysm and show the lungs to be clear except for a diagonal streak of platelike atelectasis on the right, not uncommon in a patient who has been confined to bed.

Six days after discharge, *Mr. Schock* is wakened from a nap by sudden, severe, frightening, recurrent chest pain. He is rushed back to his local hospital where his blood pressure is found to be 80/60. The electrocardiogram has not changed. What is happening to *Mr. Schock*? Please turn to *Part C, page 60,* for his second emergency chest film.

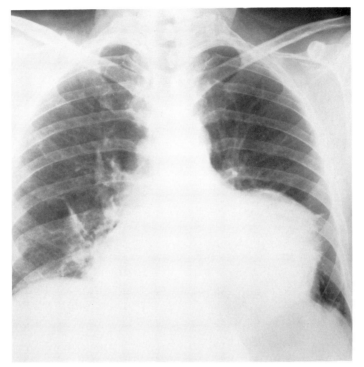

FIG. 33

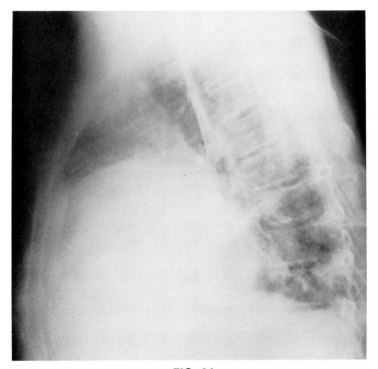

FIG. 34
FIGURES 33 & 34. Mr. Schock's discharge films

Phoenicia Figtree: (*Continued from page 15*) *Ms. Figtree's* clinical presentation strongly suggests a diagnosis of pulmonary neoplasm. A most disturbing sign is her persistent wheeze which is localized to the left chest. A wheeze is produced by narrowing in the tracheobronchial airway. In asthmatics it is generalized, temporary, and produced by bronchoconstriction. *Ms. Figtree's* persistent wheeze suggests mechanical narrowing of a bronchus in the left chest. A bronchial adenoma may do this, although bronchogenic carcinoma is a very likely diagnosis with this patient's smoking history.

Her chest films are reproduced in *Part C, page 72*. Are they consistent with your clinical diagnosis of a bronchogenic carcinoma?

Tussy Pachooka: (*Continued from page 11*) The most likely diagnosis is gastroenteritis. However, the history of bloody mucus must alert you to the possibility of an intussusception. After starting intravenous fluids you send the patient to radiology for supine and upright plain films of the abdomen. What do you think these films might show you?

Continued Part C, page 79.

Luke Stein: (*Continued from page 12*) *Dr. Stein* presents with classic symptoms and signs of a ureteral calculus. You request a stat urinalysis to confirm the presence of hematuria. The urine is clear. However, the laboratory quickly reports that the sediment contains 50 to 70 red blood cells per high-power field. Only a few white blood cells are seen. The emergency intravenous urogram which you now request is reproduced in *Part C, page 62*. What is your opinion of it?

Amanda Kent: (*Continued from page 5*) WBC: 12,400, normal differential. Sputum smear: few gram-positive diplococci, but no polys.

Chest film: There is an infiltrate on the left which on the PA film (Fig. 35) blurs the left hemidiaphragm but does not obscure the heart border and is therefore in the left lower lobe. This is confirmed on the lateral view (not shown).

Did you notice the air bronchogram visible behind the heart on the PA film? This implies that the bronchi are patent and well-aerated (Fig. 36).

You diagnose a left lower lobe pneumonia, probably pneumococcal, and relieve *Sergeant Kent* from duty, sending her to her quarters with penicillin and terpin hydrate, to return to clinic in 3 days. Please turn to *Part C, page 53*.

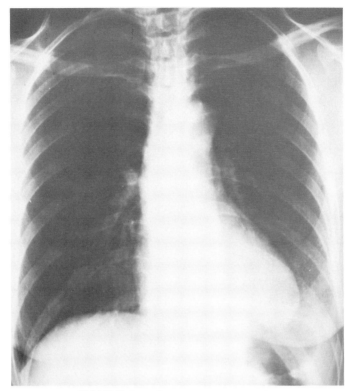

FIGURE 35. Sgt. Kent's chest film

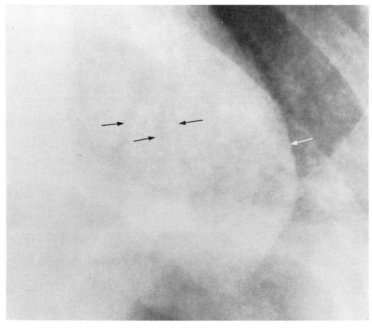

FIGURE 36. Kent's detail film — air bronchogram in left lower lobe (black arrows); heart margin (white arrow)

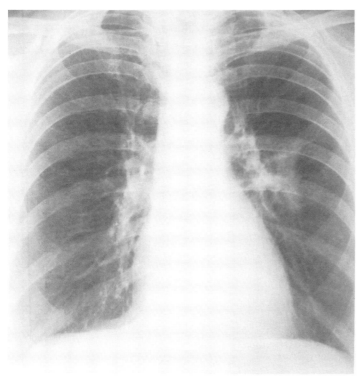

FIG. 37

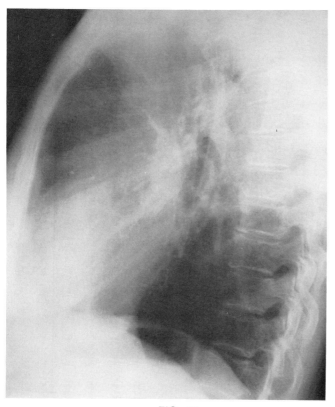

FIG. 38

FIGURES 37 & 38. Lucy's abnormal chest films

Lucy Rouge: *(Continued from page 4)* There is a patchy density in the superior segment of the left lower lobe. It is best seen on the PA view, but can also be located behind the cardiac silhouette on the lateral view. This does not have the sharp margins of a well-defined mass, but it is more localized than most pneumonias. Could it be a cancer? It could, but there are no signs of tumor metastases such as hilar adenopathy, elevation of the hemidiaphragm (which may be seen when the phrenic nerve is invaded by hilar tumor). The heart, great vessels, and thorax are normal.

The sputum culture produces only a few pneumococci and normal throat flora. Stains for acid-fast bacilli are negative as are sputum cytologies. Serum chemistries including liver function tests are normal. *Mrs. Rouge* remains afebrile and her white count remains normal. How will you proceed? Please turn to *Part C, page 68.*

Pierre Claude Tordu: *(Continued from page 17)* You send the patient to radiology for routine chest films (negative) and for supine and upright films of the abdomen. Here is the supine film (Fig. 39). What and whither?

Continued Part C, page 83.

B–41

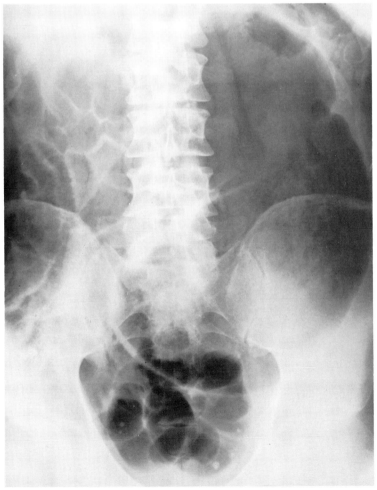

FIGURE 39. Pierre Tordu's supine film

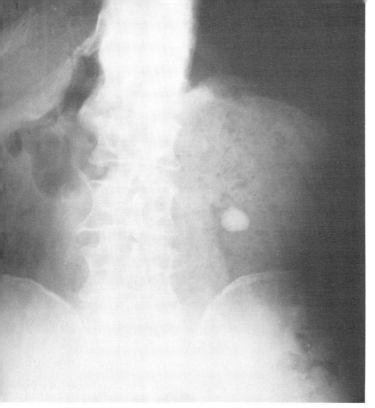

FIGURE 40.   Captain Solent's abdomen

Henry Mountjoy Solent: *(Continued from page 7)* A supine film of the abdomen is obtained (Fig. 40). It probably would have been best to include an upright film as well, but none was taken. However, there is confirmation of your physical findings. What do you see, and what do you do now?

Continued Part C, page 59.

John Gaunt: *(Continued from page 14)* Had the radiologist carried out that request for a barium enema, your patient might well have died. It is most unlikely, however, that the radiologist would have accepted your request for the enema after seeing the plain film, even if you had failed to give him the clinical history. For the film is characteristic of toxic dilatation of the colon and a barium enema is contraindicated in the face of that diagnosis (see Fig. 9, page 43).

Toxic dilatation is one of the most dreaded complications of ulcerative colitis — and it may occur at any time during the course of chronic disease, or it may represent the initial episode in an acute, fulminating case. Because of its anterior position as the patient lies supine, the transverse segment of the totally atonic colon shows the most striking dilatation. A careful look at the film will show the nodular protrusions of hyperplastic mucosa into the air-filled lumen of the transverse colon. The colon in this omi-nous condition is hugely dilated, very thin, diffusely ulcerated, and hemorrhagic, and may show areas of actual necrosis. Since the diagnosis can be made from the history, the clinical findings and the plain film of the abdomen, a barium enema is not only unnecessary but may well perforate this extensively diseased, thin-walled colon, and the patient may expire from overwhelming peritonitis.

As a matter of fact, look at the film again. Did you notice that *Mr. Gaunt's* colon was *already* perforated even at the time this film was made? The general radiolucency above the transverse colon, particularly in the region of the hepatic flexure and surrounding the stomach, represents free intraperitoneal air. Had an enema been done, the barium would have poured into the peritoneal cavity and added still further contamination to that already caused by spillage of blood and stool.

End of Case

Page 42

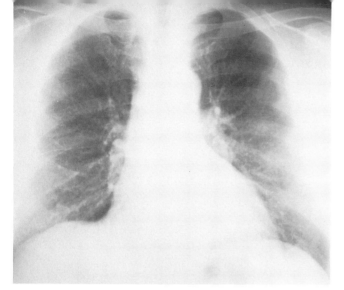

FIGURE 41.   Dollface's chest

Dollface Davenport: *(Continued from page 16)* You refer *Dollface* for a chest x-ray and laboratory examinations, and send him home with a temperature chart. When he returns in 5 days his blood tests, including BUN and blood sugar, liver function tests, and his electrocardiogram are all normal. His tuberculin skin test is strongly positive. Unfortunately, his urine culture is lost. Here is his chest film (Fig. 41).

The chest film suggests left ventricular hypertrophy. The pulmonary parenchymal markings are slightly increased and irregular, suggesting some fibrosis, but there is no evidence of active cardiopulmonary disease. How will you proceed? Please turn to *Part C, page 78.*

B–43

Repeat of FIGURE 9. Gaunt's abdomen reprinted

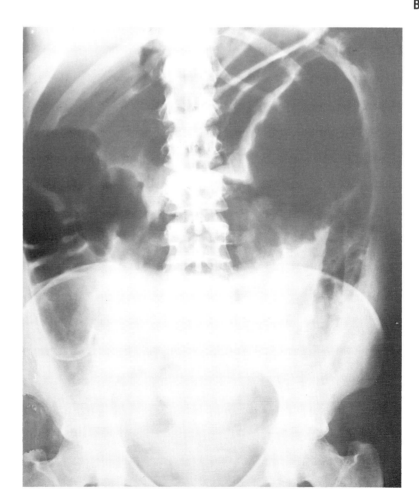

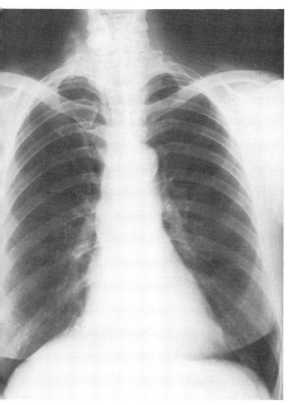

FIGURE 42. Violet's PA chest film

Violet Bloomer: *(Continued from page 7)*
This is a normal PA chest film (Fig. 42). The lateral view was also normal.

The 15 minute film from the pyelogram (Fig. 43) shows no visible function on the right and a large left kidney measuring 16.5 cm in long axis. The left kidney may be large because it is a solitary kidney or because it has gradually hypertrophied in response to diminished renal function on the right. The history of right flank pain suggests that the latter possibility is the more likely.

What additional laboratory data will you request? Blood sugar, creatinine, and urine cultures are normal. Electrolytes and urine VMA, sodium and potassium are also normal, but probably need not have been obtained, since the IVP points so strongly to hypertension of renal origin.

What will be the next step in your work-up? Please turn to *Part C, page 69.*

FIGURE 43. Violet's IVP

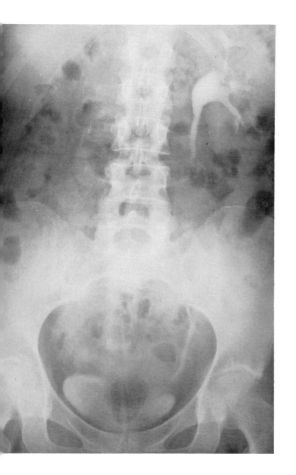

Tai Foon: *(Continued from page 2)* You should have made 3 observations: (1) there is diffuse gaseous distention of the colon, (2) there is a suspicious soft tissue density in the region of the hepatic flexure, and (3) there is a striking lack of gas or fecal material in the rectosigmoid and rectal ampulla. What diagnostic procedure would you consider doing next?
Continued Part C, page 69.

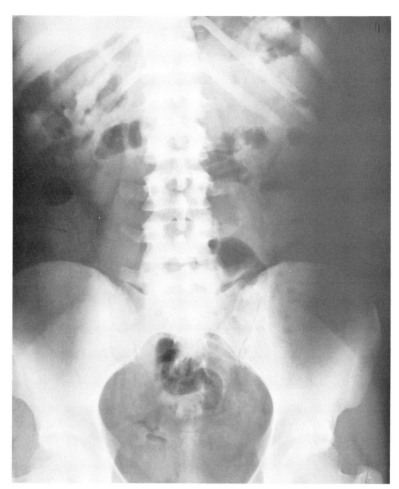

FIGURE 44. Miss Feld's abdomen

Hannah Feld: *(Continued from page 8)* Your initial request is for a supine film of the abdomen (Fig. 44). The soft tissue landmarks seem normal. Nothing is seen in the right lower quadrant . . . or is there? There is no intra-abdominal calcification to suggest an appendolith. Recurrent appendicitis is still a possibility, though, since only about 10 per cent of patients with acute appendicitis show a calcified appendiceal fecolith on x-ray.

What about the pattern and distribution of intestinal gas? There is a loop of mildly dilated small bowel in the mid-abdomen. And what about the right lower quadrant? Look again. Is there something there, or is your eye pulled back to that region because there is nothing there?

Continued Part C, page 55.

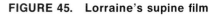

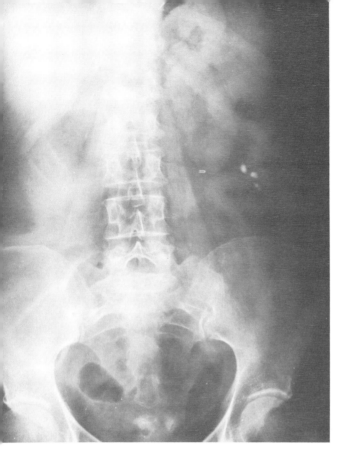

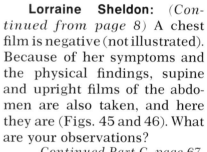

FIGURE 45. Lorraine's supine film

Lorraine Sheldon: *(Continued from page 8)* A chest film is negative (not illustrated). Because of her symptoms and the physical findings, supine and upright films of the abdomen are also taken, and here they are (Figs. 45 and 46). What are your observations?

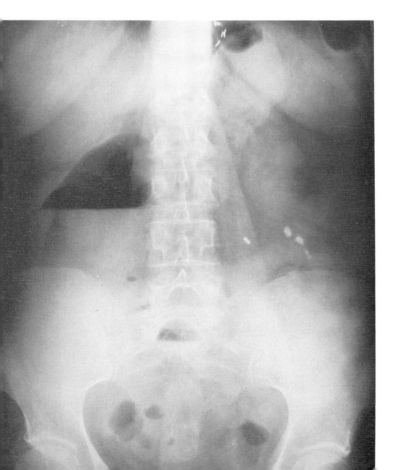

Continued Part C, page 67.

FIGURE 46. Lorraine's upright film

Jack Eveready: *(Continued from page 5)* This is *Mr. Eveready's* admission chest film (Fig. 47). The lungs may be slightly overinflated, but this is a normal chest film. The lateral was also normal. *Jack's* liver function tests are as follows (normal values are in brackets): Bilirubin direct/total: 0.6/2.0 (0.4/1.0); SGOT: 115 (40); alkaline phosphatase: 8.4 (4.0). The gall-bladder was not visualized after two consecutive days of oral contrast material. (This is what is meant by a "double dose cholecystogram"; a double dose is *not* twice the usual dose on the same day.)

What do you think is the cause of his jaundice? How can you be sure? Please turn to *Part C, page 56.*

What do you think is the cause of his jaundice? How can you be sure? Please turn to *Part C, page 56.*

B–47

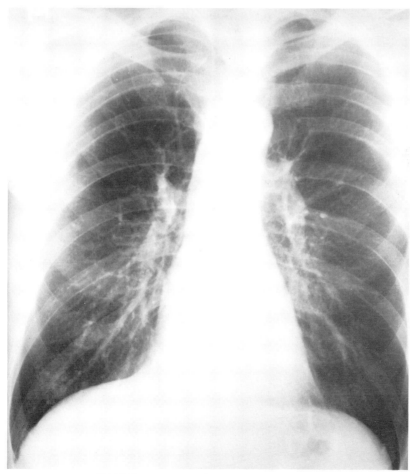

FIGURE 47. Jack Eveready's chest film

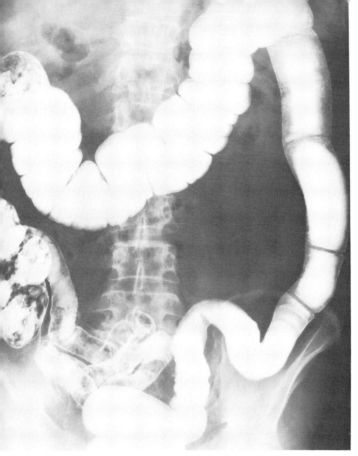

FIGURE 48. Mme. Vermilion's barium enema

Colette Vermilion: *(Continued from page 16)* Because the visualized blood is coming from higher up in the colon than can be reached by the sigmoidoscope (which means beyond the rectosigmoid-sigmoid junction), it will be necessary to ask the radiologist to do a barium enema. You must be sure to alert him to your finding of blood so that he will know that you do not consider this just another routine examination. The radiologist will then do a study specifically tailored to this patient's problem, which is obscure bleeding.

You schedule the appointment and give the patient instructions for bowel preparation, and the barium enema is done. Here are two of the films from that study (one with the colon full of barium and the other taken after the patient evacuated the enema) (Figs. 48 and 49). The radiologist contacts you and says that he is not satisfied with the examination on 2 counts: (1) the colon was not adequately cleaned of fecal material to allow proper visualization of the interior of the bowel and (2) the films were not perfectly centered to the patient with the result that a portion of the right colon is never seen on any of the 5 films which were actually obtained. He concludes that although he has seen "no gross lesion," he does not feel the study warrants reassurance that the colon is negative for small polypoid filling defects. Now what do you do?

Continued Part C, page 57.

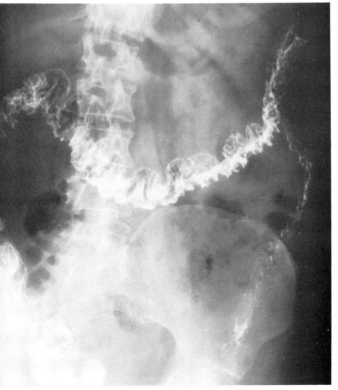

FIGURE 49. Post-evacuation film

Caleb P. Salem: *(Continued from page 4)* There is a patchy infiltrate on the right (Fig. 50), best seen on the lateral view (Fig. 51) where it appears as a wedge-shaped density, narrower than you would expect the middle lobe to be. The hemidiaphragms are flattened and there may be some linear scarring at the bases. The heart and great vessels are normal.

The history and chest film are consistent with an acute right middle lobe pneumonia in a smoker with chronic bronchitis. The middle lobe atelectasis could be due to poor ventilation secondary to the acute inflammation superimposed on chronic bronchitis, or to a mucus plug, but you must also consider a tumor. How will you proceed? Would you have biopsied the axillary node? Remember, the lymphatics of the lung do not drain to the axilla. The node showed only chronic inflammation.

Please turn to *Part C, page 71.*

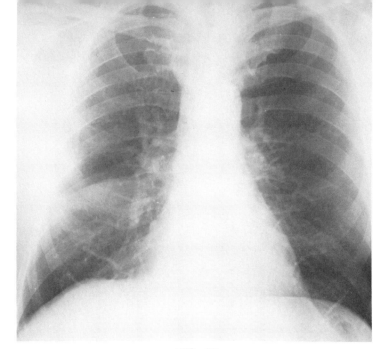

FIG. 50

B-49

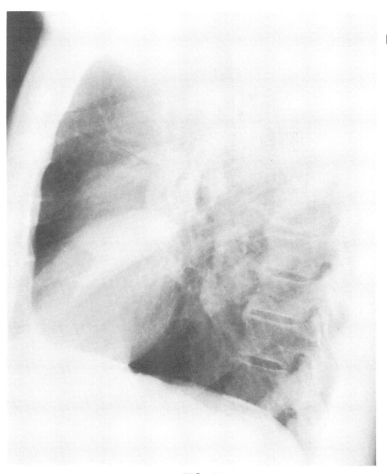

FIG. 51
FIGURES 50 & 51.   Caleb's chest films

PART C

PART C

Nicky Arachis: *(Continued from page 25)*
We hope not. Any child in whom inhalation of a foreign body is possible from the history should have inspiration/expiration films. The bronchus normally dilates during inspiration and narrows during expiration. When a foreign body interferes with egress of air from one lung, air will be "trapped" on the obstructed side and there may be demonstrable mediastinal shift at expiration as the nonobstructed lung empties. Any single PA chest, so ordered, will be obtained at full inspiration, when, indeed, the mediastinum may be in midposition.

Figure 53 is *Nicky's* expiration film. Compare the 2 studies, and the drawings below.

Obviously there is mediastinal shift at expiration, and there must be a (nonopaque) foreign body in the left main bronchus with air trapping behind it. A peanut *(Arachis hypogaea)* was recovered at bronchoscopy. Had you let this child go home, he might well have developed atelectasis and infection in the obstructed lobe before the correct diagnosis could be established.

End of Case

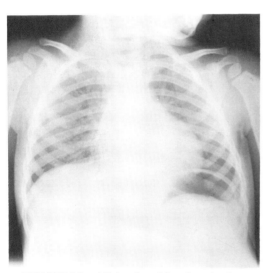 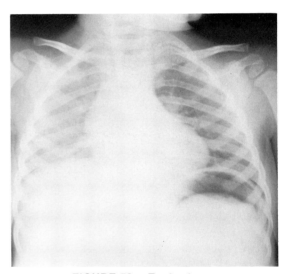

FIGURE 52. Nicky Arachis—Inspiration   **FIGURE 53. Expiration**

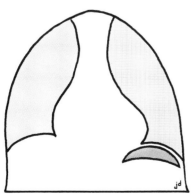 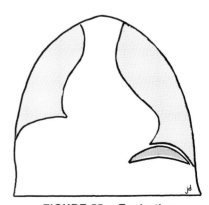

FIGURE 54. Inspiration   **FIGURE 55. Expiration**

Amanda Kent: *(Continued from page 38)* Two weeks later *Sergeant Kent* finally returns. She is no better and still has sticky rales on the left side. The sputum culture grew out normal throat flora. Here is her repeat chest film (Fig. 56).

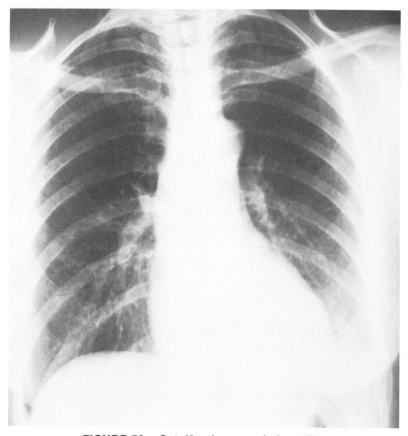

FIGURE 56. Sgt. Kent's second chest film

There has been no improvement in the chest film. If anything, the infiltrate is a little more dense. You go through the history again. The cough is worse at night. There is scant sputum and it is watery, never pink. *Sergeant Kent* thinks she is a little short of breath now, but has not had any fevers, chills, or sweats. No one in her section is ill. She has no pets. Her last overseas tour was to Germany 3 years ago.

What are you considering for a diagnosis now? Please turn to *Part D, page 86.*

Alfred Stevens: *(Continued from page 22)* Careful examination will allow you to exclude peripheral lymphadenopathy. Don't forget to examine the adenoidal and tonsillar areas of the hypopharynx.

If Hodgkin's disease spreads from the mediastinum, it often involves the spleen and para-aortic lymph nodes. These areas can be examined only in-directly. Figure 57 shows the tip of a spleen of normal size. Figure 58 is a representative film from the IVP which showed no displacement of the ureters by para-aortic lymph nodes.

How can you better examine the ab-dominal lymphatics? Please turn to *Part D, page 92.*

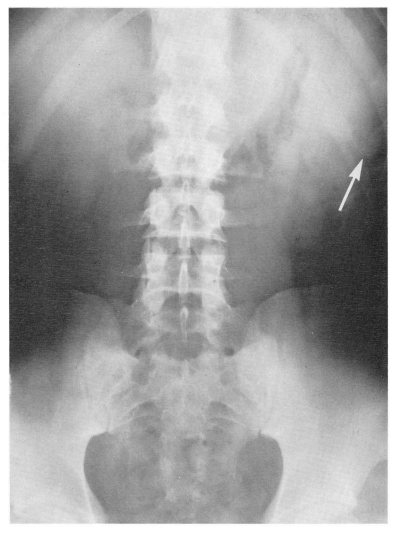

FIGURE 57. Alfred Stevens' abdomen

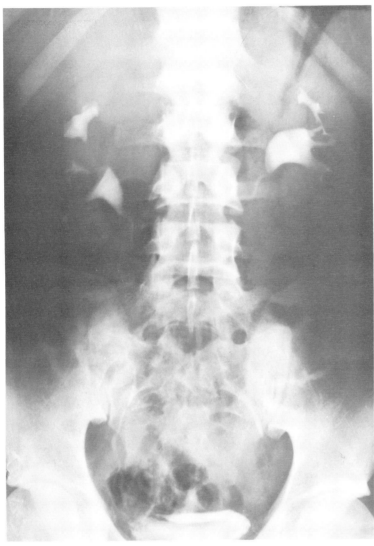

FIGURE 58. One film from Stevens' IVP

Hannah Feld: *(Continued from page 45)* If you are suspicious of the overall "grayness" of the right lower quadrant, and the lack of bowel gas in this area—you are right. What should you suspect? A tumor could cause this, displacing air-filled bowel away from the area. An inflammatory mass or an abscess in this region, causing irritation of the lower psoas muscle on the right and pain on hyperextension of the leg could also account for the x-ray and physical findings. Since the urinary tract was not suspected as a primary source of the patient's symptoms, it was elected to omit an intravenous pyelogram. Instead, on the chance that the patient might have appendicitis, a barium enema was considered. Would you request that study on this patient?

Continued Part D, page 96.

Jack Eveready: *(Continued from page 47)* Although there must be some liver necrosis with an elevated SGOT, this value is not very high. The alkaline phosphatase is disproportionately increased suggesting obstructive jaundice. The preponderance of conjugated bilirubin and decreased urine urobilinogen suggest the same thing. Does the failure to visualize the gallbladder mean that Jack has cholecystitis?

No. With a bilirubin of 2.0, there may be enough liver or bile duct dysfunction to prevent an uninflamed gallbladder from being visualized. However, with a bilirubin under 4.0, it may still be possible to visualize the gallbladder and common duct by giving the contrast intravenously and obtaining laminographic cuts through the area of the porta hepatis. Here is *Mr. Eveready's* intravenous cholangiogram (Figure 59 with *drawing*, Figure 60).

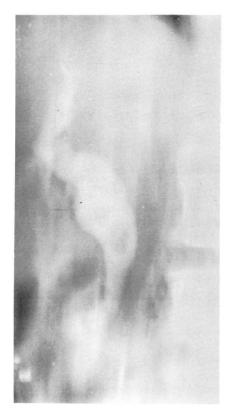

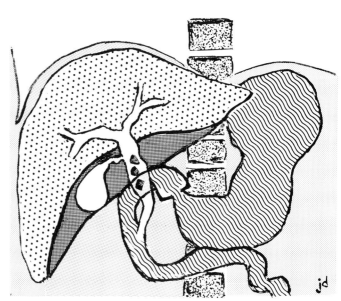

FIG. 59   **FIG. 60**
FIGURES 59 & 60.   Eveready's intravenous cholangiogram

You can see, to the right of the spine, dilated intrahepatic bile ducts and several lucent areas in the distended common duct. These were proved at surgery to be biliary calculi. Please turn to *Part D, page 88.*

Colette Vermilion: *(Continued from page 48)* Have the enema repeated! Since the standard bowel preparation (including castor oil on the night before the barium enema) apparently did not clean this patien's colon, you should reschedule the study and this time put *Madame Vermilion* on a special bowel preparation. One method of doing this is to place her on a low-residue diet for 2 days and on an all-liquid diet during the final day before the study. Also, she should take milk of magnesia for 2 nights and then castor oil on the afternoon before the barium enema.

This is done, and here is one film from the repeat study (Fig. 61). See anything?

Continued Part D, page 90.

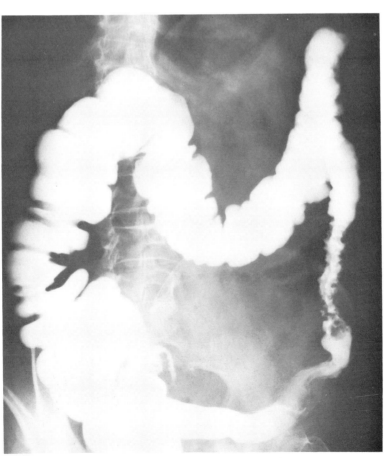

FIGURE 61.   Mme. Vermilion's second enema

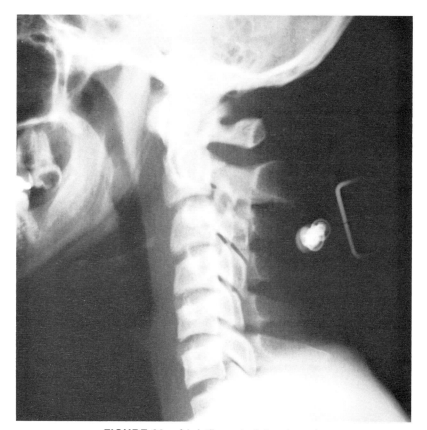

FIGURE 62. Lightfinger's lateral neck

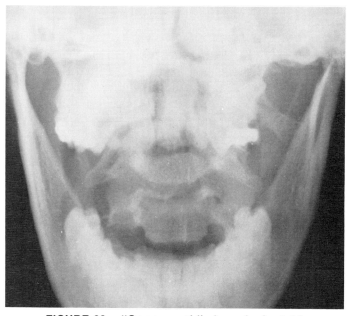

FIGURE 63. "Open mouth" view of odontoid

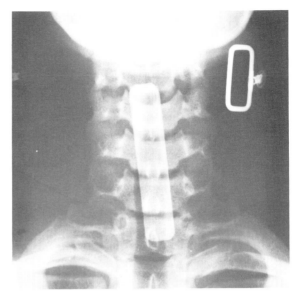

FIGURE 64.   AP neck

Clyde Lightfinger: (*Continued from page* 23) The retropharyngeal soft tissues visualized on the cross-table lateral view (Fig. 62) should make you very suspicious of a fracture of the upper cervical spine. There is an increase in the width of the soft tissue shadow between the pharyngeal airway and the anterior aspect of the upper 4 cervical vertebrae, suggesting a retropharyngeal hematoma. Normally this distance is only 3 mm in the adult. Here it measured more than 10 mm.

Instead of a normal lordotic curve there is straightening of the cervical spine with slight subluxation of C2 anteriorly on C3. The arrow on the detail film of this same view (Fig. 65, next page) points to a C2 pedicle fracture. No other fractures are seen on this view; the odontoid appears intact. Posteriorly there are metallic densities, part of the collar.

No abnormalities are seen on the AP view (Fig. 64). After several attempts at open mouth views (Figure 63 is an example), the odontoid is still not adequately visualized in the AP projection. You cannot rule out a fracture of this structure from the lateral film alone. How will you visualize the odontoid in the AP projection without subjecting the patient to unnecessary manipulation?

Continued Part D, page 105.

C-59

Henry Mountjoy Solent: (*Continued from page* 42) The plain film of the upper abdomen shows a large calcified left renal calculus, unrelated to *Solent's* present illness. The entire left side of the abdomen shows a mottled appearance, suggesting a large amount of food and fluid in the stomach.

Would you next proceed to an upper G.I. series? If so, what do you expect to find?

Continued Part D, page 108.

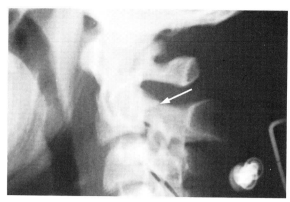

FIGURE 65. Lightfinger—detail of second cervical vertebra

Maximilian Schock: *(Continued from page 36)* Does this help you? What are your tentative diagnoses (Fig. 66)?

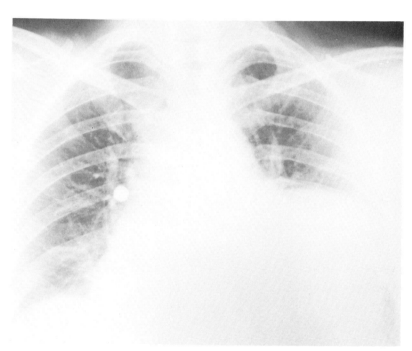

FIGURE 66. Mr. Schock's second emergency chest film

Certainly severe chest pain and shock 20 days after a documented myocardial infarction make you consider the possibility that the infarction has extended into the adjacent myocardium. However, in this special case of an aneurysmal left ventricular wall, a more serious possibility exists. The ischemic myocardium may have become so necro-

tic that it is leaking. The aneurysm does look a little larger, but one cannot be sure, because this is a portable film.

Mr. Shock's family doctor feels that immediate cardiac surgery may be necessary, so he sends the patient in an ambulance to your University Hospital. How will you evaluate and treat him? Please turn to *Part D, page 111.*

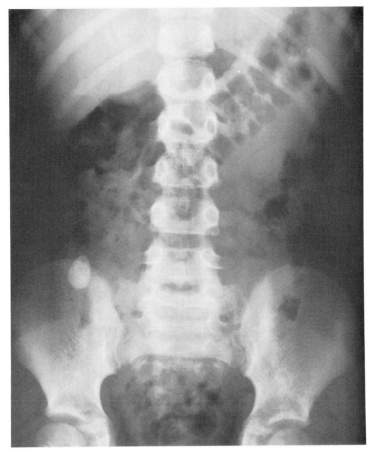

FIGURE 67. Penny's plain film

Penny Stone: *(Continued from page 24)* Both abdominal films (the supine film is supplied, Fig. 67) reveal a pear-shaped, laminated, calcific density measuring nearly 2 cm in length in the right lower quadrant. No other abnormalities are seen. This calcification is classic in configuration for a large appendiceal fecalith (or appendolith). It lies lateral to the right ureter and inferior to both the right kidney and the usual position of the gallbladder. This finding supports a diagnosis of chronic appendicitis. Even prophylactic appendectomy has been recommended in asymptomatic patients with this radiographic finding because there is increased incidence of appendicitis and perforation.

The urinalysis is normal. There is no evidence of a urinary tract infection. The white count is elevated to 16,500 with 69 per cent polys and 10 per cent band forms. The nurse informs you that *Penny's* rectal temperature has risen to 101° F. What is your diagnosis *now* and how will you confirm it?

Continued Part D, page 107.

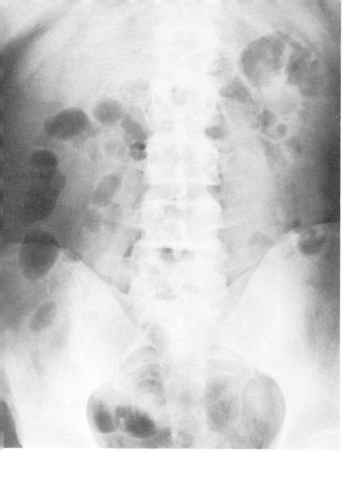

FIGURE 68. Stein's preliminary film

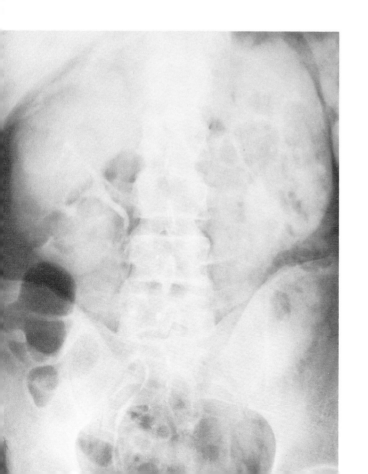

FIGURE 69. 5 minute film

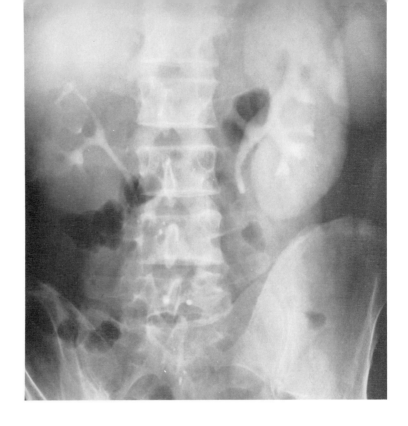

FIGURE 70. 60 minute film

Luke Stein: *(Continued from page 38)*
The plain film (Fig. 68) reveals mild
splenomegaly, residual contrast within
the subarachnoid space of the lumbo-
sacral spine from a previous myelogram,
and phleboliths in the right pelvis. No
calculus is seen overlying the left urinary
tract; are you surprised?

Of course not. *Dr. Stein* may have a
lucent stone which cannot be seen on the
plain film. Evidence for such a stone in
the left ureter is suggested by the 5
minute film (Fig. 69). No contrast is
seen in the left calyces at this time. This
finding is compatible with diminished
left renal excretion secondary to ureteral
obstruction. Ureteral stones usually
produce partial obstruction because they
are frequently spiculated, allowing small
amounts of urine to flow around them.

A lucent stone can usually be visualized when contrast reaches the site
of obstruction. On the 60 minute film
(Fig. 70), the ureter is found to be obstructed at the level of the L3 to L4 interspace. Note the expected mild dilatation
of the left intrarenal collecting system
and proximal left ureter, reflecting elevated pressure within this system.

The intense left nephrogram (Fig.
70) results from hyperconcentration of
contrast. The collecting system is obstructed, but the left kidney continues
to function. Water reabsorption from the
obstructed tubules hyperconcentrates
the fluid within them.

All these radiographic findings are
classic for a lucent left ureteral stone.
Lucent stones, which comprise about
20 per cent of ureteral stones, usually
consist of uric acid crystals. *Dr. Stein*
passed his ureteral stone spontaneously
while voiding and it has been lost. You
request a serum uric acid level as well
as a 24 hour urine collection for uric
acid excretion rate. The serum level is
normal, but the urinary excretion rate is
significantly elevated. You start him on
allopurinol.

Are you satisfied with the appearance
of the right kidney?

Continued Part D, page 103.

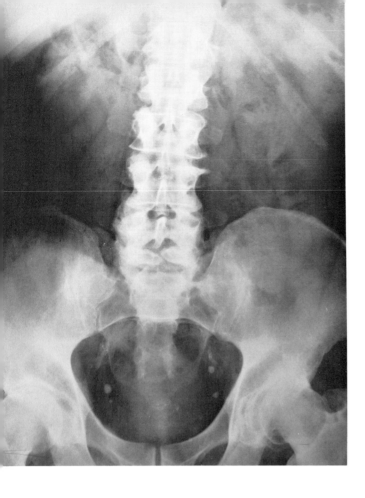

FIGURE 71. Waters' preliminary film

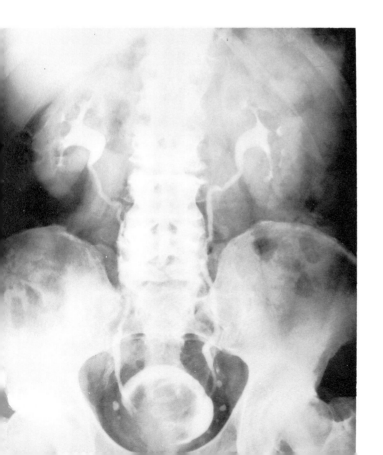

FIGURE 72. Waters' IVU

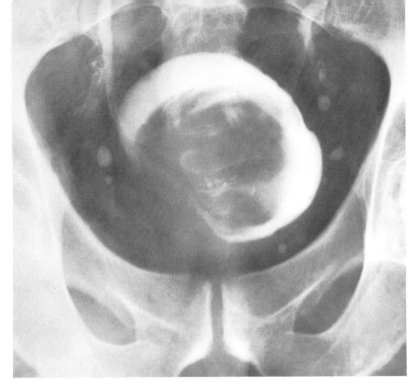

FIGURE 73. Detail of bladder

Ernest Waters: *(Continued from page 26)*
The chest films are normal, without evidence of tuberculosis. No radiopaque renal calculi are seen on the plain abdominal film (Fig. 71), although there are several incidental findings, including degenerative arthritis of the left hip, as well as vascular calcifications and phleboliths in the pelvis. To be certain that none of the phleboliths are distal ureteral calculi, compare the plain film with the contrast film (Fig. 72). All the calcifications are external to the urinary tract.

The contrast film shows normal kidneys and ureters with normal renal function demonstrated bilaterally. In the bladder (Fig. 73), however, there is a large, round, lobulated filling defect which is nearly completely surrounded by a rim of contrast. The appearance is typical of a pedunculated bladder tumor, most likely carcinoma, which is attached to the right bladder floor by a thick pedicle. The bladder wall is thickened

and flattened at the site of attachment, suggesting that the tumor is infiltrating the wall. The irregularities along the left dome of the bladder are also consistent with malignant infiltration. Frequently bladder tumors will obstruct a ureteral orifice, producing hydroureter and hydronephrosis, although this did not occur here.

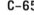
C–65

The appearance of bladder tumors may be mimicked by large blood clots and rarely by nonopaque stones within the bladder, as well as by a collection of gas in the rectum, which may be seen through a normal contrast-filled bladder in the AP projection.

Benign tumors infrequently occur in the bladder. Secondary tumors arise by direct extension from the prostate gland, bowel, uterus, cervix, and ovary. How will you confirm your diagnosis of a primary bladder carcinoma?

Continued Part D, page 87.

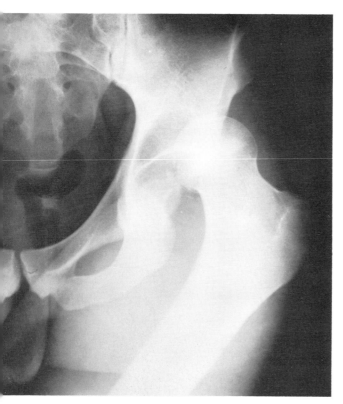

FIGURE 74. Jay's hip

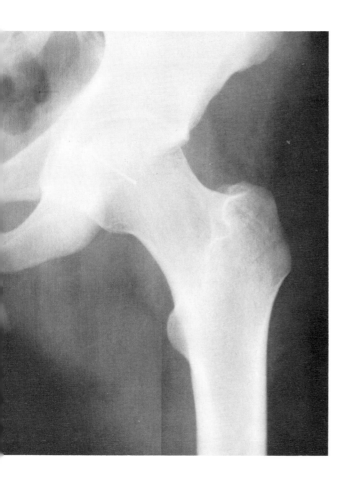

Jay Roach: *(Continued from page 33)* A detail of the pelvic film (Fig. 74) shows a posterior dislocation of the left hip and a bone fragment underlying the left femoral head consistent with an acetabular rim fracture. In posterior dislocation, the femoral head lies at a higher level than the acetabular roof and lateral to it. Consequently the involved leg will be adducted on physical examination. With anterior dislocation, the femoral head usually overlies the obturator foramen with the limb abducted. No abnormalities are observed on the chest, abdomen, or skull films (not illustrated).

The admission hematocrit is 45 per cent. Urinalysis is normal. Analgesics are administered, and the patient is scheduled for hip surgery in the morning. He remains stable during the night and serial hematocrits show no evidence of blood loss. At surgery, a small fracture of the left acetabular rim is confirmed. The dislocation is reduced and the fracture fragment is fixed with a short piece of metallic wire (Fig. 75). Postoperatively you start the patient on anticoagulants and he does well.

On the second postoperative day *Mr. Roach* complains of increasing right upper quadrant pain. You note marked spasm and guarding in the right upper quadrant. No bowel sounds are heard. What diagnostic possibility are you considering, and how will you proceed?

Continued Part D, page 109.

FIGURE 75. Jay's post-op film

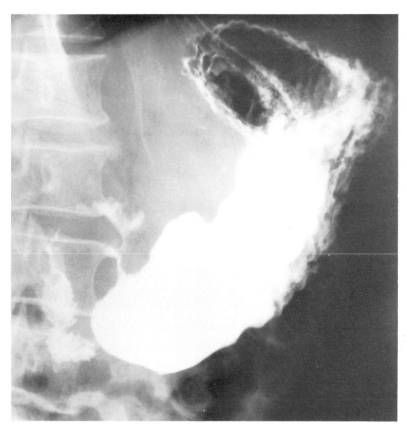

FIGURE 76. Watling's stomach

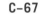

Carlton Watling: (*Continued from page 28*) You slowly aspirate about half of the remaining gastric contents and then allow the patient to sober up, under careful observation. When he is less restless, he is connected to constant gastric suction and treated with electrolyte replacement, IV fluids, and mild sedation for 3 days. You now send him back to radiology for evaluation of the cause of his acute gastric obstruction. Here is a representative film from his upper G.I. series (Fig. 76). Your diagnosis?

Continued Part D, page 107.

Lorraine Sheldon: (*Continued from page 46*) The films show several calcified mesenteric lymph nodes in the left abdomen. Vagotomy clips are noted about the distal esophagus (and one surgical clip near the lymph nodes) from her previous partial gastrectomy. There is marked distention of the right colon with gas, as seen on the supine film. On the upright film, the gas in the right colon has risen into the hepatic flexure and the air-fluid level indicates that the ascending colon also contains fluid. There is an ominous lack of gas in the transverse and descending segments of the colon. What do you do next?

Continued Part D, page 104.

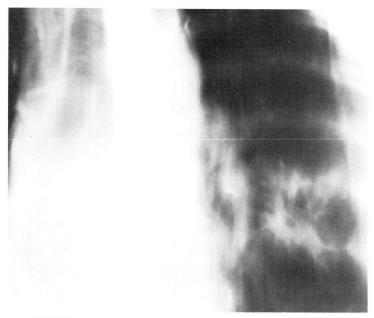

FIGURE 77. Laminographic cut of Lucy's left lower lobe

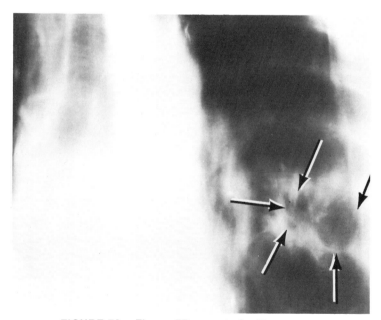

FIGURE 78. Figure 77 repeated with arrows

Lucy Rouge: *(Continued from page 40)*
There are several ways to better visualize
the abnormal lung. Fluoroscopy was performed and was of no help. Here is a
representative film from a series of
laminographic cuts through the lesion
(Figs. 77 and 78).

The patient is slightly rotated. You
can see the tracheobronchial air column
to the right of the spine. The lesion has
a relatively lucent center surrounded by
a density radiating out from it. No definite mass can be seen. There may be a
cystic area just distal to the main lesion.
What are your tentative diagnoses, and
what is your plan? Turn to *Part D, page
89.*

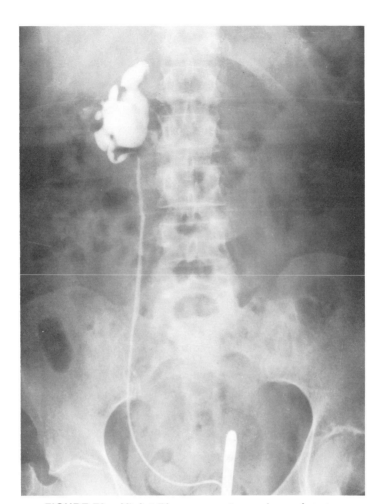

FIGURE 79. Violet Bloomer—retrograde pyelogram

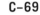

Violet Bloomer: *(Continued from page 44)* As you see, a retrograde pyelogram was obtained (Fig. 79): both kidneys are present. The right renal pelvis is dilated but the ureter is of normal caliber. The proximal ureter is deviated medially. This almost certainly represents hydronephrosis due to obstruction of the proximal ureter. Will you obtain an arteriogram?

Please turn to *Part D, page 91.*

Tai Foon: *(Continued from page 44)* Since the abrupt ending of the colonic distention in the lower bowel suggests that there may be an obstruction at this point, sigmoidoscopy should be done next. You do this procedure and find that the rectal ampulla is indeed empty, but there is a fungating tumor high in the rectosigmoid. Would you now proceed to do a barium enema?

Continued Part D, page 87.

Cecily Mannerborn: *(Continued from page 34)* The PA film of the chest shows what at first appears to be a high left hemidiaphragm. On closer inspection, you note that the apex of the dome of this "diaphragm" is shifted laterally and that there is blunting of the left costophrenic angle. On the lateral film of the chest, the elevated "left hemidiaphragm" shows a ski-slope anterior margin. Also, the posterior gutter on the left is blunted. These findings suggest infrapulmonary pleural effusion (fluid in the interpleural space, elevating the lung base and conforming to the curve of the hemidiaphragm). The anterior slope of the fluid, as seen on the lateral film, is due to the infrapulmonary fluid abutting against the underside of the major fissure on the left (Fig. 80). The physical findings on examination of the chest are confirmed and explained.

As for the abdomen, incidental observations first: the metallic clip superimposed over the pelvis is on a sanitary belt. The faint radiopaque densities and small calcified plaques in the buttocks, best seen in the soft tissues just lateral to and above the right acetabulum, are due to past intramuscular injections. Did you make the really significant observations on this supine film of the abdomen? First, there is no obvious pancreatic calcification (which may sometimes be seen in patients with chronic pancreatitis). Secondly, there is a very suspicious soft tissue density in the left upper quadrant of the abdomen which constricts the upper part of the gastric air bubble. Is there a tumor in the stomach — or is there something pressing against the stomach from outside and distorting it?

What x-ray methods are available to help you in further evaluating this area? Which one have you decided to request first and why?

Continued Part D, page 106.

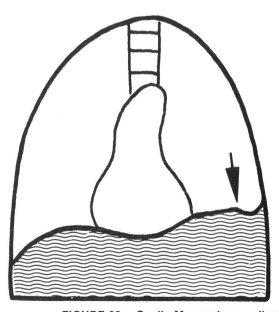 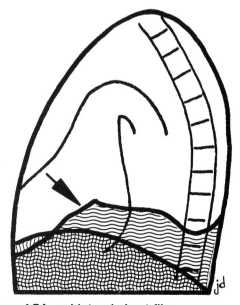

FIGURE 80.   Cecily Mannerborn — diagram of PA and lateral chest films

Caleb P. Salem: *(Continued from page 49)* You smear and culture the sputum which is presumably coming from the abnormal lung. As the initial sputum samples contain many diplococci, you start *Mr. Salem* on penicillin. This eradicates the pneumococci, and after 5 days the sputum contains normal throat flora, but the chest film does not improve. What next?

Bronchoscopy should show you the right middle lobe bronchus as well as the orifices of the first branches and will allow you to obtain a good sputum sample. However, no abnormality is seen at bronchoscopy. There is no blood coming from the affected lobe and the sputum is once again negative for pathogens including fungi and tuberculosis. Cytology is also negative. *Caleb* is afebrile and feeling better. What will you do? Please turn to *Part D, page 93.*

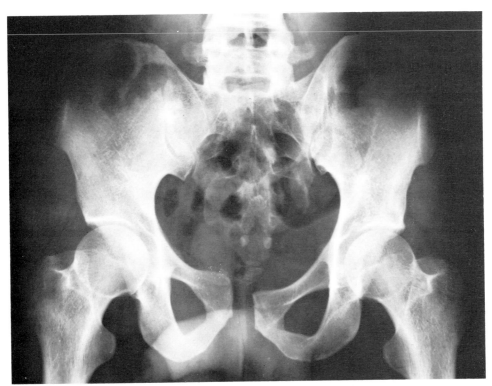

C-71

FIGURE 81.   Chester's pelvis

Chester Winston Wilcox: *(Continued from page 31)* The pelvis film (Fig. 81) shows a dislocated, "burst" pelvis. There are no fractures, but there is diastasis of the pubic symphysis from ligamentous trauma associated with a subluxed or "sprung" left sacroiliac joint. Note the increased width of the left sacroiliac joint when compared with the right. The chest and abdomen films are unremarkable (not shown).

The laboratory reports a urinary sediment with 50 to 60 red blood cells per high-power field. The hematocrit is 45 per cent. *Mr. Wilcox's* vital signs are remaining stable.

Which radiographic studies will you request now? What do you expect them to show?

Continued Part D, page 98.

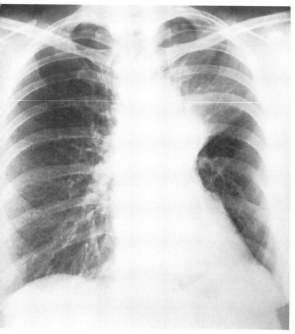

FIG. 82

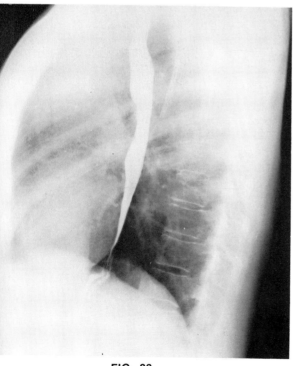

FIG. 83
FIGURES 82 & 83.   Ms. Figtree's chest

Phoenicia Figtree: *(Continued from page 38)* The PA film (Fig. 82) shows a smooth rounded left hilar mass just inferior and lateral to the arch of the aorta. This film also demonstrates the classic features of a left upper lobe collapse. There is a ground-glass density in the left upper lung field which represents the atelectatic left upper lobe. The density of the lobe is increased because it contains less air. This decrease in volume of the left upper lobe is accompanied by elevation of the left hemidiaphragm and slight mediastinal shift to the left. Notice that the right heart border overlies the spine on this well centered film instead of lying lateral to it.

The radiologist on duty does fluoroscopy of the chest after seeing this PA film. He observes normal excursions of both hemidiaphragms without evidence of paralysis on the left. Therefore, the left phrenic nerve is not involved by tumor. The left hilar mass is observed to pulsate.

He gives *Ms. Figtree* barium in order to search for compression of the esophagus by the hilar mass or by adjacent nodes. Films are then taken with barium in the esophagus. No esophageal compression is observed. The lateral film (Fig. 83) shows obliteration of the normal retrosternal anterior clear space by the overlying density of the collapsed left upper lobe.

Since the left hilar mass has been observed to pulsate, you must differentiate it from aorta. The pulsations could either be transmitted or represent expansile pulsations of the mass itself. Which study would you request now?

Continued Part D, page 97.

Pat and Mike: (*Continued from page 31*) We are not pulling your leg; this really happened. The extra piece of bone was removed from *Mike's* foot and replaced in *Pat's* femur with the help of an intramedullary rod. Figure 84, made 6 weeks later, shows excellent healing. Both patients have made good recoveries. The piece of bone was sterilized with radiation before being restored to its owner. Garlands to anyone realizing that a clinically short leg has not been accounted for if there is no overriding of fragments. In addition, of course, the ends of the bones in the first film do not actually match in shape.

End of Case

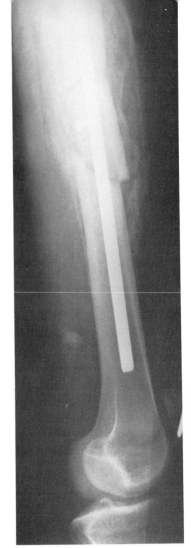

FIGURE 84. Pat's femur   C-73

Adalena Cardoza: (*Continued from page 32*) The plain film shows numerous calcifications apparently located in the kidneys. Their crowded appearance on the left suggests that the left kidney is small. The pyelogram that follows (Fig. 85) shows blunted and crowded calyces and loss of cortex indicating pyelonephritis in that kidney. At the same time the laboratory results show BUN 30, serum calcium 12.5, and serum phosphorus 2.1. What next?

Continued Part D, page 100.

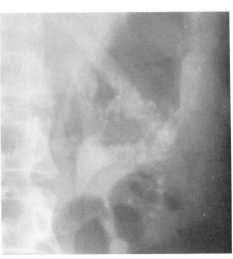

FIGURE 85. Adalena's pyelogram

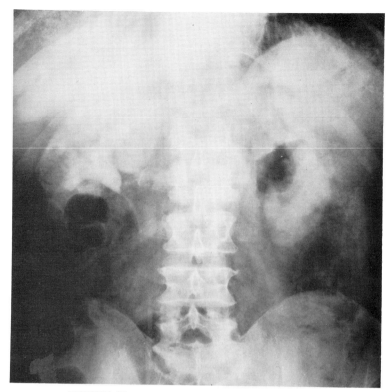

FIGURE 86.   5 minute film from Rocco's IVU

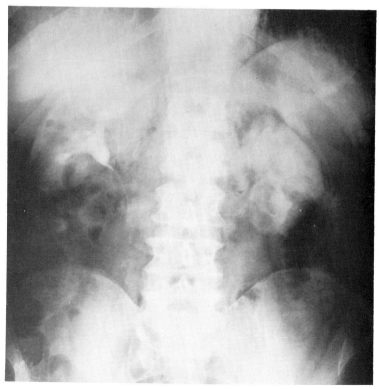

FIGURE 87.   2 hour film

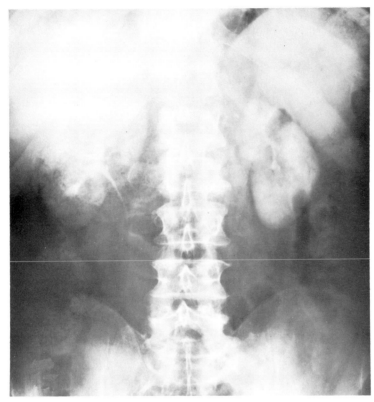

FIGURE 88. 4½ hour film

Rocco Malatesta: *(Continued from page 23)* You are, no doubt, struck by the significant difference in size between the two kidneys. The right measures 13.0 cm in length, the left only 9.5 cm. The earliest films are not reproduced here, since renal function is so diminished on the left that the nephrogram is not demonstrated until 5 minutes (Fig. 86) and contrast is not seen within the left calyces until 4 and a half hours (Fig. 88).

With a lesser degree of diminished function, the delayed appearance of contrast may be demonstrated only on the films made prior to 5 minutes in a hypertensive study.

Mr. Malatesta's chest film shows slight left ventricular enlargement, consistent with the presence of hypertension, but is otherwise unremarkable. (It is not reproduced here.) The plasma cortisol and urine VMA are reported as normal. There is no chemical evidence for diabetes and the urine culture is negative.

What are the diagnostic possibilities now, and how will you proceed?

Continued Part D, page 101.

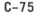 C–75

Vittorio Antonini: *(Continued from page 26)* His hematocrit is reported as 34, not surprising if he does have thalassemia. You re-examine the boy and are again impressed with the tenderness in the left upper quadrant. You cannot discount the possibility of splenic rupture—yet. What additional procedures are available to you?

Continued Part D, page 110.

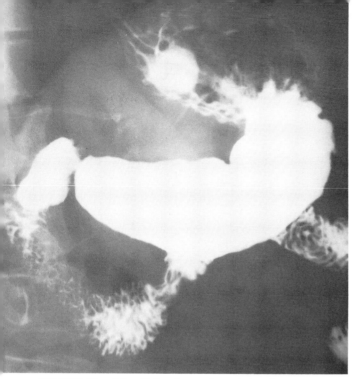

FIGURE 89. Ninette's stomach and duodenum

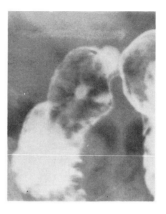

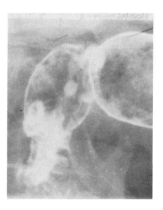

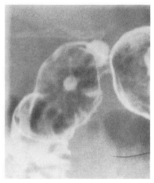

FIGURE 90. Spot films
of duodenal bulb

Ninette de Gautière: *(Continued from page 30)* "Emergency upper G.I. series. Acute bleeder. Duodenal ulcer?" Next telephone the radiologist to arrange personally for this study, and then send the patient to x-ray with an attendant and orders for frequent checking of vital signs.

The custom-tailored barium study for the acute upper G.I. bleeder is a limited one, carried out with special precautions against initiating fresh hemorrhage. The patient is given very little barium; no palpation is used, and no pressure spot films are made. Barium itself has been shown to be quite harmless and this type of limited study is perfectly safe if the radiologist is informed about the patient. Knowing that he has an acute bleeder to study will also enable him to schedule this patient before others with less pressing problems. Although the colon may be studied eventually, a barium enema is not indicated at this time.

What do you make of *Ninette's* films? Figure 90 shows *Miss de Gautière's* ulcer crater in the as-yet-not-deformed duodenal bulb which is ballooned out with air. These spot films were obtained with *Ninette* positioned right side up so that air flowed from the stomach into the elevated duodenal bulb. The ulcer is not visualized on the prone film of the stomach (Fig. 89) because this film was obtained at the end of the examination, after the patient had been given more barium to drink.

Ninette remains stable and does well on a medical regimen.

End of Case

Mary Pastone: (*Continued from page 25*) Films of the spine certainly show pronounced bone loss. Note that in the lateral view the density of the vertebral bodies is not much greater than that of the soft tissues anterior to them. The intervertebral discs seem to be expanding at the expense of the bony end plates of the bodies of the vertebrae. No lytic areas are seen but one lumbar vertebra looks collapsed. (Calcification is noted within a widened abdominal aorta.)

You make a presumptive diagnosis of osteoporosis.

Two weeks later, *Mrs. Pastone* returns to the emergency room with a fracture of the humerus near the elbow, which occurred spontaneously when she lifted a heavy frying pan. With this history and with the discovery of anemia, you decide to admit her for study.

What will you request?

Continued Part D, page 95.

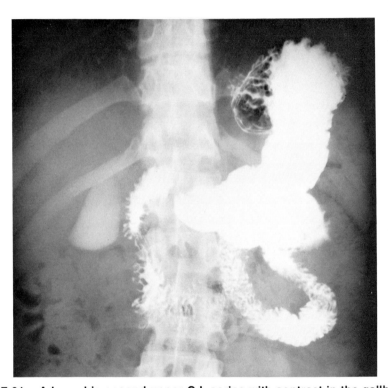

C-77

FIGURE 91. Adumreb's second upper G.I. series with contrast in the gallbladder

Dr. Notlimah Adumreb: (*Continued from page 26*) Several studies are possible, but because of the patient's right upper quadrant discomfort, you elect to do an oral cholecystogram next. This is normal. The following day a repeat upper G.I. series is done (Fig. 91). What do you see?

Continued Part D, page 94.

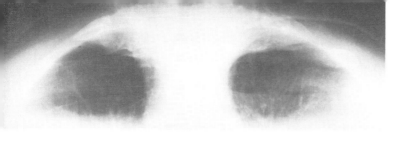

FIGURE 92. Apical lordotic view—
Davenport

Dollface Davenport: (*Continued from page 43*) Having documented the fever and obtained most of the initial laboratory data, you admit *Mr. Davenport* to the hospital, repeat his urine culture, and begin obtaining periodic blood cultures. What are your tentative diagnoses?

Even today, recurring fevers without focal symptoms have a high probability of being tuberculous in origin. *Mr. Davenport* has a strongly positive tuberculin skin test and some evidence of chronic lung disease. Figure 92 is the apical lordotic view. There is no definite scarring and certainly no infiltrate or cavity to suggest active tuberculosis.

Nevertheless, you culture the urine for tuberculosis and obtain an intravenous pyelogram (Fig. 93). The IVP shows no distortion of renal architecture (pyelectasis or loss of renal cortex), which would be expected from the scarring of chronic renal infections. Nor is there any deviation of the ureters as is sometimes caused by enlarged para-aortic lymph nodes in lymphoma.

The urine culture and 2 of the 4 initial blood cultures are growing out a gram-negative rod tentatively identified as Salmonella. What now? Please turn to *Part D, page 87*.

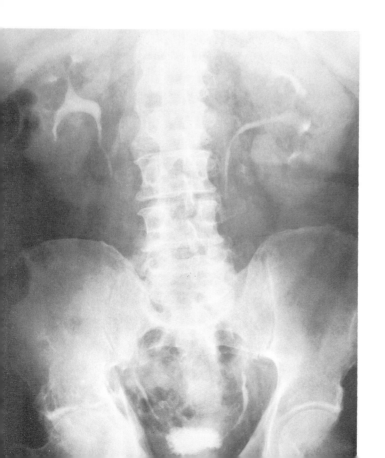

FIGURE 93. Davenport's IVP

Tussy Pachooka: *(Continued from page 38)* The erect film showed no free air or abnormal fluid levels. Here is the supine plain film (Fig. 94). Does it help you?

Continued bottom of page.

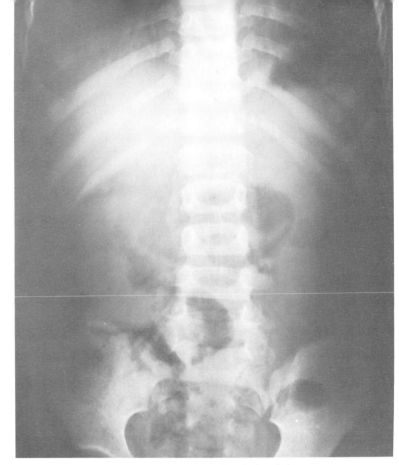

FIGURE 94. Tussy Pachooka's abdomen

C-79

Ruby Hobson Reingold IV: *(Continued from page 24)* The illness which caused Ruby to see her family doctor 2 weeks ago sounds like a Mycoplasma pneumonia. Cold agglutinins are strongly positive. A tuberculin skin test is negative. Liver function tests to evaluate the possibility of widespread metastatic tumor are normal.

Renal cell tumors spread via the renal vein into the bloodstream and may present as asymptomatic lung masses, though they usually present with hematuria. Because of the red cells in *Mrs. Reingold's* urine, an IVP is done. It is normal.

You have not yet precisely localized this lesion. At fluoroscopy, it was not possible to separate the nodule from the diaphragm. How can you get a better view of the mass?

Turn to *Part D, page 109.*

Tussy Pachooka *(Continued from above)* Yes, there *is* a round soft tissue mass on the right side of the abdomen between the 12th rib and the iliac crest. The scattered gas shadows tell you nothing except that there is no roentgen evidence of intestinal obstruction. The presence of a mass with her history is very suggestive of intussusception, usually ileocolic in a young child. What will you do next?

Continued Part D, page 99.

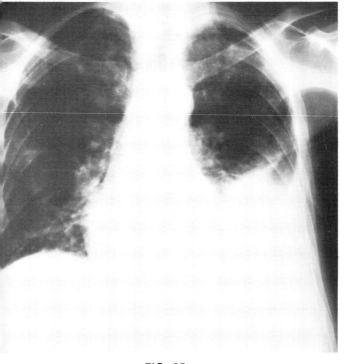

FIG. 95

Johnny Walker: *(Continued from page 33)* The chest films (Figs. 95 and 96) show the left pleural effusion which you predicted from the physical examination. The heart does not appear to be enlarged. That tubular density overlying the chest on the PA projection is an IV line.

Gross ascites is seen on *Mr. Walker's* abdomen film (Fig. 97). There is a ground-glass appearance throughout the abdominal cavity with loss of the parenchymal organ outlines.

You perform a diagnostic left thoracentesis. Cytology reports malignant cells. Which studies would you request now and what do you expect them to show?

Continued Part D, page 102.

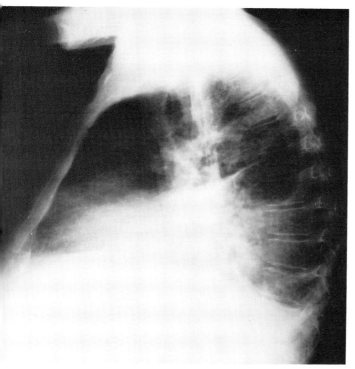

FIG. 96
FIGURES 95 & 96. Johnny Walker's PA and lateral chest films.

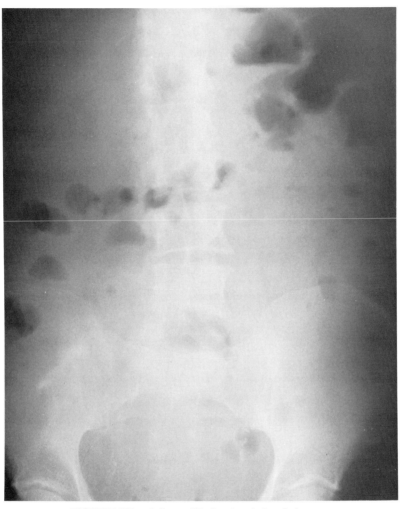

FIGURE 97. Johnny Walker's plain abdomen

Roberto Yglesias: *(Continued from page 32)* Whether this is a primary bone tumor or a metastasis from tumor elsewhere, the fracture must be immobilized. This will require open reduction and fixation with an intramedullary rod. You should biopsy the tumor at the time of surgery. The pathologist may be able to give you an idea of the tumor's site of origin and its radiosensitivity. If it is a radiosensitive tumor, you may want to irradiate the area of the fracture.

If the tumor is completely undifferentiated, you still have statistics to help you. Most solitary bone tumors in this age group are metastatic. Lung, kidney, thyroid, and, in females, breast are the most common sources of lytic metastases. These areas are easy to examine clinically or radiologically.

In the presence of metastases, a cure is usually not possible, but you should still look for the primary site. Further metastases or direct spread from an untreated primary lesion may considerably shorten the patient's remaining life or cause unnecessary misery from pain and disability.

Mr. Yglesias' primary lesion was a squamous cell carcinoma of the lung.

End of Case

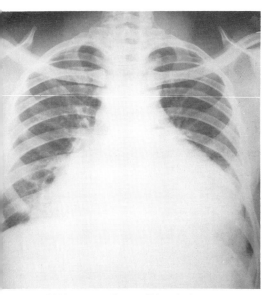

FIGURE 98. Corey Bloat's heart

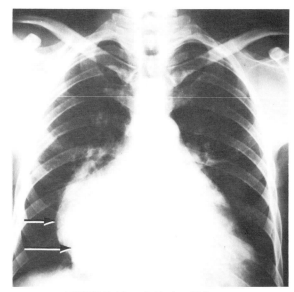

FIGURE 99. A "mitral" heart
(Top arrow is margin of left atrium; bottom arrow is margin of right atrium)

Corey Bloat: *(Continued from page 30)* Large formless cardiac silhouettes usually result from one of three things: pericarditis with pericardial effusion; myocarditis or myocardiopathy, including ASCVD; or valvular disease, especially mitral regurgitation. In the first situation there is a more or less normally beating heart inside a sac of fluid. In the second case, the entire myocardium may be flabby and weakened, whereas in valvular disease one chamber is usually more altered in structure than another. The radiographic (and EKG) differentiation of the 3 processes depends on demonstrating these differences.

Of course, you also have more clinical information to help you. In this instance rheumatic heart disease is un-

likely; the disease would have been symptomatic long before the heart got this big. You don't see focal chamber enlargement on this film; nor was it seen at fluoroscopy. Figure 99 shows another patient's large "mitral" heart in which the giant left atrium is still producing a "double density" distinct from the right atrium which makes up the normal right heart border.

Mr. Bloat's heart, Figure 98, could conceivably be a heart dilated from myocarditis. However, when you check the blood pressure during a respiratory cycle, you find that the systolic pressure drops by 25 mm Hg on inspiration. How will you proceed now?

Please turn to *Part D, page 111.*

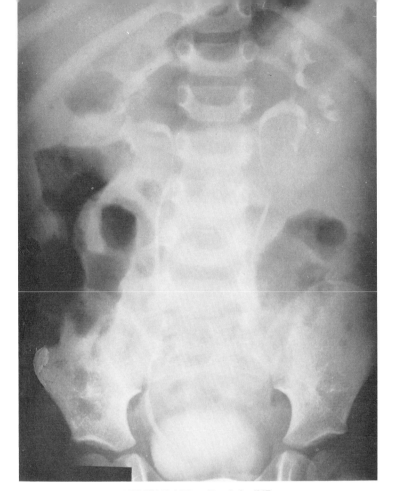

FIGURE 100.   Kevin's IVP

Kevin Somers: *(Continued from page 29)* This late film from the IVP again shows little bowel gas to the left of the spine, but it does not define a mass. It tells you that there is no mass arising from the kidneys, but also that there is no mass in the retroperitoneal space. If there were, the kidneys and/or ureters would be displaced from their normal position.

Sometimes the retroperitoneal fat outlines the kidneys and psoas margins so well on the plain film that an IVP is superfluous, but usually an IVP is the first step in evaluating a poorly localized abdominal mass. In infants the IVP is especially pertinent because hydronephrotic kidneys and Wilms' tumors make up a large proportion of abdominal masses in this age group.

What will you do next? Turn to *Part D, page 89.*

Pierre Claude Tordu: *(Continued from page 41)* The plain film of the abdomen shows some scattered gas in small bowel loops on the right side of the abdomen. There is a huge gas-filled structure occupying most of the left side of the abdomen. Some mottled densities within it suggest fecal material. What do you think has happened and what would you do next?

Continued Part D, page 94.

PART D

PART D

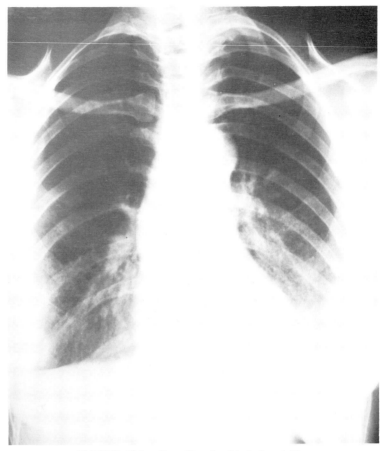

FIGURE 101. Sgt. Kent's third chest film

Amanda Kent: *(Continued from page 53)* Among other things, you should be considering a nonbacterial pneumonia, especially one due to *Mycoplasma pneumoniae.* Mycoplasma pneumonia typically presents as a continuous hacking cough with little sputum and few systemic symptoms. The chest x-ray frequently shows an unexpectedly dense infiltrate, often in a lower lobe, which may take several weeks to clear. Viral pneumonias, psittacosis, and tuberculosis may have a similar onset.

You switch *Sergeant Kent* to eryth-romycin, test the serum for cold agglutinins, and culture the sputum for tuberculosis. Once again she fails to return to your clinic. When she does, 6 weeks have passed, the cough is no better, she has persisting clear sputum, and she is short of breath. Here is her chest film (Fig. 101).

The left lower lobe infiltrate is unchanged, and now there is pleural fluid and thickening on the right. What is your next step? Please turn to *Part E, page 125.*

Dollface Davenport: (*Continued from page* 78) With this many positive cultures, you are not dealing with a contaminant and start *Dollface* on chloramphenicol. The problem now is to find the source of the infection. Moreover, before a week is out, you find that even though the salmonella is sensitive to your drug *in vitro*, the fevers are continuing. There are still no focal symptoms.You know that salmonella often lodges in the gallbladder, spine, or a diseased area of the cardiovascular system. Now you remember *Mr. Davenport's* history of backache. Please turn to *Part E, page 118.*

Tai Foon: (*Continued from page* 69) Really, no further x-ray studies are indicated. A barium enema will only confirm what you have already seen and even if barium could be passed beyond the tumor in order to visualize the rest of the colon, it would be unwarranted, since the patient might not be able to evacuate it all and he would then have a barium impaction added to his problem.

The only other serious diagnostic possibility from the plain film of the abdomen would be acute diverticulitis with obstruction, but that is excluded by the history, the absence of fever, or laboratory signs of inflammatory disease, and the sigmoidoscopic examination. Surgery is indicated.

At operation, there is indeed an obstructing carcinoma of the rectosigmoid. Segmental resection and a primary anastomosis are done. At the same time, a colotomy of the hepatic flexure is carried out and a bulky lipoma removed which was responsible for the suspicious density seen on the plain film.

End of Case

D-87

Ernest Waters: (*Continued from page* 65) At cystoscopy you observe that the patient has a large tumor almost completely filling the bladder. Biopsy is interpreted as squamous cell carcinoma, much less frequent than transitional cell carcinoma in this organ.

Bone series and liver scan are negative for metastatic disease. A radical cystectomy with pelvic lymph node dissection is performed; an ileal loop is created as a urinary diversion. Postoperatively, the patient does well and is discharged on the 19th day.

Six months later, *Mr. Waters* returns complaining of malaise, weakness, and lumbar back pain. He has lost 20 lbs and looks cachectic. What complications are you considering? Which studies will you request?

Continued Part E, page 116.

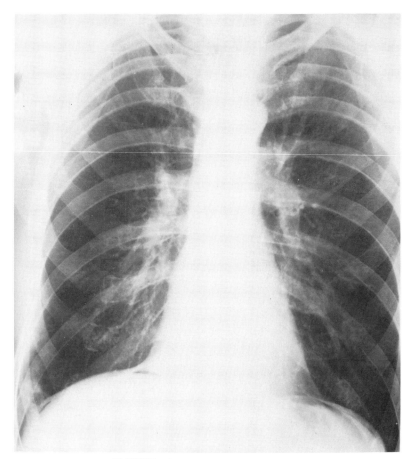

FIGURE 102. Jack's post-op film

Jack Eveready: *(Continued from page 56)* Jack's first post-op day was uneventful, but the next day he developed a low-grade fever and leukocytosis associated with pleuritic chest pain. Here is his chest film (Fig. 102). What do you see?

The air under the diaphragm is not abnormal for a post-op patient, but that patchy density in the right costophrenic angle was not on the admission film. It does not have the linear configuration of platelike atelectasis and it should, with this history, suggest a pulmonary embolus. However, the rest of the chest is unchanged. The heart sounds are unchanged, as is the electrocardiogram. What will you do now? Remember that the LDH and white count may both be abnormal in a patient recovering from biliary surgery. Please turn to *Part E, page 122.*

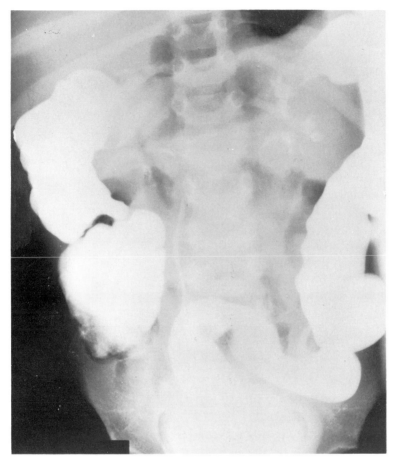

FIGURE 103. Kevin Somers

Kevin Somers: *(Continued from page 83)* The barium enema, performed immediately after the normal IVP, is also normal (Fig. 103). The complete study showed no extrinsic or intrinsic filling defect and no displacement of colon from its normal position. What now?

Turn to *Part E, page 119.*

Turn to *Part E, page 119.*

Lucy Rouge: *(Continued from page 68)* This is a common problem. You know this lesion wasn't present a year ago when the previous Board of Health film was obtained, but cancers can easily grow this big in a year. The lesion looks like a cavity, not a mass, but lung tumors, especially squamous cell tumors, may cavitate or there may be an abscess cavity distal to an endobronchial lesion. A bronchogram may help in that differential, but is not done. Bronchoscopy is performed. It shows purulent material coming from the superior segmental bronchus of the left lower lobe. Cultures of this material produce a mixed flora. Cytologic studies are negative. Would you operate now? Please turn to *Part E, page 121.*

Please turn to *Part E, page 121.*

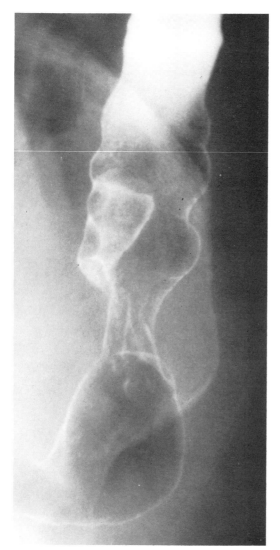

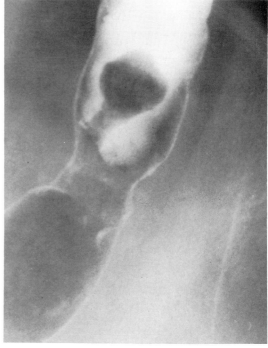

FIG. 104   **FIG. 105**

FIGURES 104 and 105.   Mme. Vermilion

Colette Vermilion: *(Continued from page 57)* Yes, you do. There is a very suspicious filling defect in the distal descending colon. It measures about 1.5 cm in size and may well be a polyp. The radiologist saw it too and he immediately did an air contrast examination. This is a refined procedure, which is usually done right after a regular enema in cases of obscure bleeding, or when a suspicious defect is seen in a colon which otherwise appears to be clean of fecal debris. Here are 2 spot films from the air contrast enema (Figs. 104 and 105). They show a definite polyp on a short stalk. Should you recommend to your patient that she have surgery for its removal—or is this a type of polyp which you believe could be safely watched and restudied in 6 months or a year?

Continued Part E, page 114.

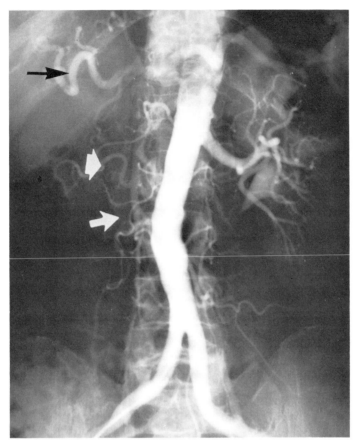

FIGURE 106. Violet's aortogram (Black arrow, hepatic artery; white arrows, lumbar collaterals)

The aorta and visualized main branches including the left renal artery are normal. The right renal artery is not seen. Instead there are several moderately enlarged lumbar vessels extending into the region of the right renal bed.  These presumably are collateral blood supply to the unvisualized renal remnant. *Mrs. Bloomer's* right renal vein renin level is elevated.

At surgery you find a thrombosed aberrant right renal artery crossing the right ureter. The nubbin of renal tissue that remains shows chronic pyelonephritis and hydronephrosis. Presumably the aberrant vessel caused the hydronephrosis and pyelonephritis which progressed to thrombosis of the right renal artery.

Following nephrectomy, *Mrs. Bloomer* becomes normotensive.

End of Case

Violet Bloomer: *(Continued from page 69)* Not long ago, this patient would have been operated on without an arteriogram. Nowadays arteriography is usually performed in order to give the surgeon a better idea of the abnormal anatomy and so that the renal veins can be catheterized to assay renin levels. How do you interpret this aortogram (Fig. 106)?

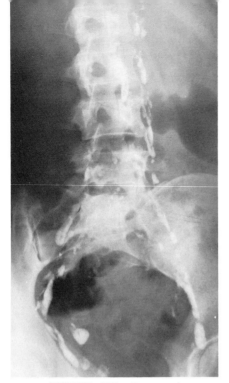

FIGURE 107. Stevens' lymphangiogram

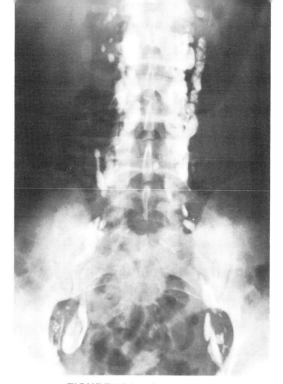

FIGURE 108. An abnormal lymphangiogram

Alfred Stevens: *(Continued from page 54)* A lymphangiogram will outline these nodes. In this procedure, 15 cc of oily contrast are slowly injected into the lymphatics of the feet and followed fluoroscopically as the contrast gradually flows up the lymphatic chains of the leg and abdomen to the thoracic duct. Figure 107 is one film from *Mr. Stevens'* normal lymphangiogram. Figure 108 is an abnormal study from another patient who has lymphoma.

The abnormal lymphangiogram shows enlarged "foamy" or "soapy" nodes with multiple filling defects. Figure 109 is a detailed view of a lymphomatous node.

Lymphangiograms are difficult to interpret. Normal lymph nodes and nodes enlarged in response to infection may look similar to nodes involved by tumor. For this reason the radiologist does not make a diagnosis on the basis of a single node and, similarly, he avoids basing his conclusions on the appearance of the inguinal nodes, since these have often been distorted by previous infections.

Would *Mr. Stevens'* normal lymphangiogram complete your work-up? Turn to *Part E, page 123.*

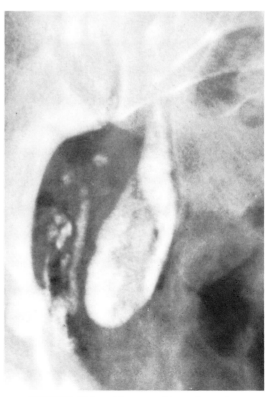

FIGURE 109. Abnormal lymph node

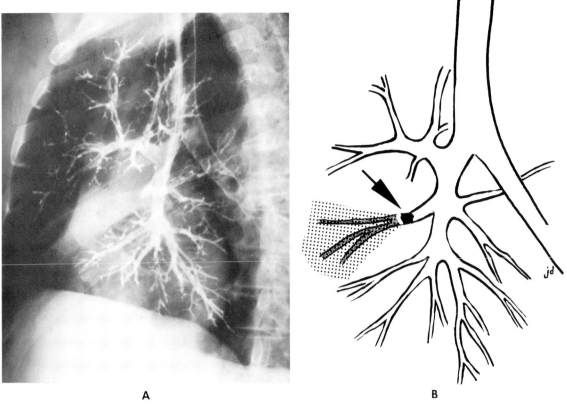

A   B

FIGURE 110A & B. Caleb's bronchogram

Caleb P. Salem: *(Continued from page 71)* If you would do a bronchogram now, we agree. In fact, *Caleb* insisted on going home and returned a month later with no change in his chest film. Here is the bronchogram obtained at that time (Fig. 110). There is a mass obstructing the bronchus to the right middle lobe. This could be a small parenchymal lesion. If this is an endobronchial lesion it could be an inflammatory mass, an impacted foreign body, or even the impression of an adjacent lymph node, but it should be considered a bronchial tumor until proved otherwise. At surgery a bronchial adenoma is found.

Bronchial adenomas are low-grade malignancies, more common in women, which arise from the bronchial mucosa and are therefore usually situated centrally near the main stem bronchi. They may cause hemoptysis, but they are usually asymptomatic until they block the bronchus and result in segmental atelectasis and/or pneumonia, as they did in *Mr. Salem*. These are relatively vascular tumors and therefore should not be biopsied through a bronchoscope. Another interesting fact about them is that the "carcinoid" type, which comprises 90 per cent of bronchial adenomas, occasionally secretes hormones. Serotonin is the most common hormone, but ACTH and insulin have also been recovered from bronchial adenomas.

End of Case

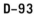

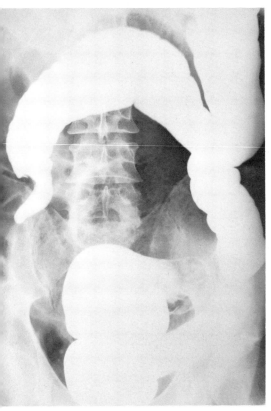

FIG. 111

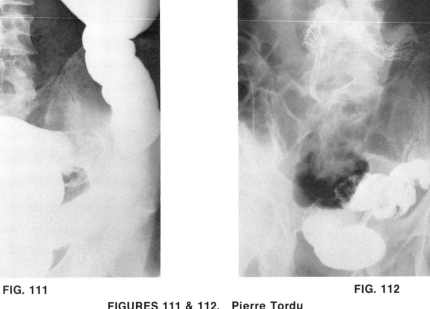

FIG. 112

FIGURES 111 & 112.   Pierre Tordu

Pierre Claude Tordu: *(Continued from page 83)* After consultation with the radiologist and without any bowel preparation, you request an emergency barium enema to confirm what you by now strongly suspect to be the diagnosis. Here are the barium enema films (Figs. 111 and 112). Were you correct?

Continued Part E, page 120.

Dr. Notlimah Adumreb: *(Continued from page 77)* The duodenal obstruction is relieved! The stomach and duodenal cap continue to look normal. Certainly no ulcer is seen. In the descending duodenum, in the area where there was almost complete obstruction on the first upper G.I. series, there are now only some mildly swollen mucosal folds. However, this segment of the duodenum curves medially, suggesting that there may indeed be a mass present pressing upon it from the lateral side. The gallbladder can still be seen opacified from the oral cholecystogram of the day before, and it is of normal size and too high to press upon the mid descending duodenum. What do you think may be wrong, and what study will you request now?

Continued Part E, page 126.

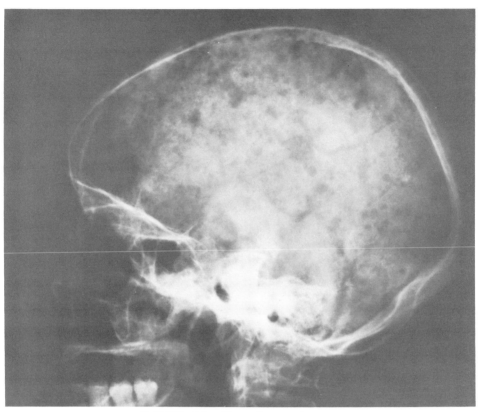

FIGURE 113.   Mary Pastone's skull

Mary Pastone: *(Continued from page 77)* Initial blood studies show her to have a severe normocytic anemia. The smear shows pronounced rouleaux formation. The laboratory also reports hyperproteinemia, serum calcium 14.8 and normal phosphorus and alkaline phosphatase.

The next day the electrophoretic pattern is returned, showing the presence of hyperglobulinemia with striking elevation of both the gamma and beta fractions. There is Bence-Jones protein in the urine and both bone marrow and the skeletal survey confirm the diagnosis of multiple myeloma. Is the lateral skull film in keeping with this diagnosis? (Fig. 113).

Yes. It is important to remember that although 90 per cent of all patients with multiple myeloma have bone pain at some time, 5 per cent never show any radiographic changes at all, and a great many smolder along with films which are indistinguishable from osteoporosis for some time before the spotty, punched-out, smooth-margined lesions that are so characteristic develop. Remember that 40 to 50 per cent of the bone must be lost before the radiologic appearance itself is very impressive. Of course the diagnosis of simple osteoporosis is excluded by finding the pathognomonic proteins of myeloma in serum and urine, *if* one thinks of looking for them. For this reason, too, patients with a tentative diagnosis of osteoporosis in this age group probably deserve a skeletal survey from time to time rather than just spine films. It is often easier to be sure of punched-out lesions in bones (like the skull and ribs) where the cortex is smooth and flat than in complex bones like the vertebrae. *Mrs. Pastone's humeral fracture was, of course, pathologic.*

End of Case

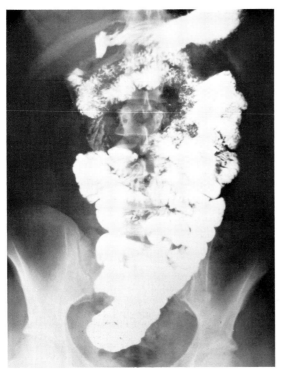

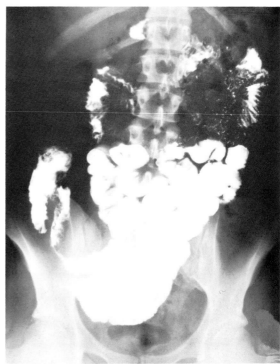

FIGURE 114. Hannah's 30 minute film   **FIGURE 115.** 60 minute film

Hannah Feld: *(Continued from page 55)* The barium enema is done because it is felt that a gentle but careful study of *Hannah's* colon, in the absence of signs of perforation and peritonitis, might be the most direct method of obtaining the diagnosis of appendiceal inflammatory disease. This would be particularly true if the barium enema showed evidence of an extrinsic pressure defect against the medial side of the cecum as a result of an inflammatory mass, and if, in addition, a thin, irregular tract of barium defined a partially filled appendiceal lumen. It was also felt that, should the barium enema be unrewarding, it would then be necessary to proceed with an upper G.I.

series and small bowel study. In such a case it would be wise to do the barium enema first to rule out such other colonic diseases as ulcerative colitis, tuberculosis, and amebiasis, all of which may affect the cecum.

The barium enema is negative and the G.I. series and small bowel study are done 2 days later. The first film (Fig. 114), taken at 30 minutes, shows barium progressing through normal jejunum into mid ileum. The right lower quadrant is still suspiciously empty. The next film, at 60 minutes (Fig. 115), shows barium in terminal small bowel and just beginning to fill the cecum. What is abnormal?

Continued Part E, page 117.

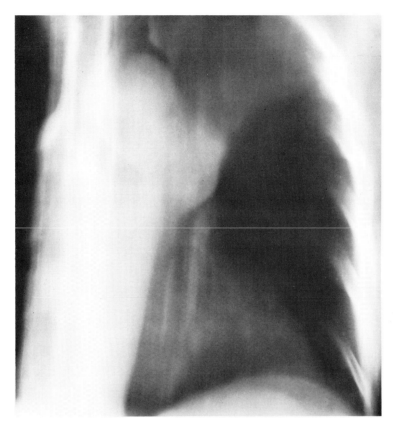

FIGURE 116. Tomogram of Phoenicia's left hilum

Phoenicia Figtree: *(Continued from page 72)* Tomography of the left pulmonary hilum is done. Several cuts (Figure 116 is an example) demonstrate a definite interface between the lateral margin of the descending aorta and the overlying left hilar mass. Thus the mass is separate from the aorta and must represent tumor. The left upper lobe bronchus could not be identified on any of the tomographic cuts and is presumably completely obstructed by tumor. This finding is expected in the presence of left upper lobe collapse.

Next, on bronchoscopic examination, you find concentric narrowing of the left main stem bronchus, the source of the wheeze. A mass is observed to protrude out of the left upper lobe bronchus. Biopsy of the mass is reported as adenocarcinoma.

End of Case

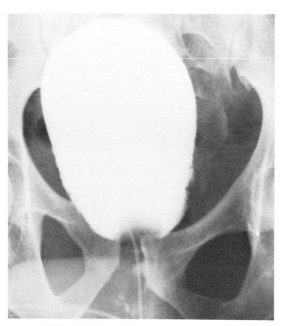

FIGURE 117. Chester's cystogram

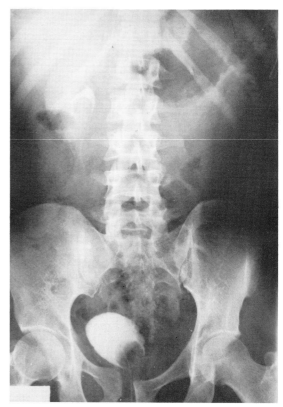

FIGURE 118. Chester's IVU

Chester Winston Wilcox: *(Continued from page 71)* Pelvic dislocations are frequently associated with rupture of the bladder or urethra, or avulsion of the urethra from the bladder. In a patient with clear urine, rupture and avulsion are unlikely. However, you request a cystogram to be certain. You also request an intravenous urogram in order to rule out left renal trauma as the cause of *Mr. Wilcox's* left flank pain and microscopic hematuria.

The cystogram (Fig. 117) shows displacement of both lateral walls of the bladder medially by bilateral pelvic hematomas. No extravasation of contrast is seen; there is no evidence of trauma to the bladder or urethra. Did you note the Foley catheter in the base of the bladder?

The intravenous urogram (Fig. 118) demonstrates a normal right kidney and right ureter, but no renal function on the left. The left kidney appears to be present. *Mr. Wilcox* denies any past history of urinary tract symptoms or disease. He has not had a nephrectomy. What is your diagnosis now and how will you confirm it?

Continued Part E, page 115.

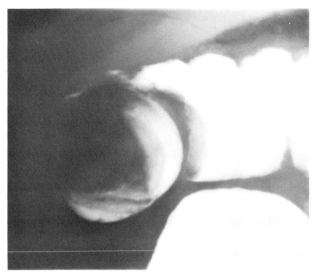

FIGURE 119. Tussy's spot film

Tussy Pachooka: *(Continued from page 79)* In intussusception, a barium enema carried out with very low pressure and no palpation may be diagnostic in showing the intraluminal mass, the intussusceptum. The barium enema may also be therapeutic, gently reducing the intussusception until the cecum and terminal ileum are seen filled with barium in their normal anatomic location in the right lower quadrant. Of course prompt surgery is the proper procedure if there are any signs of perforation or peritoneal irritation, or if the story is longer than 12 to 15 hours. But in the early or uncomplicated case, radiologic reduction has as good a record of success as surgery and no greater an incidence of recurrence. Figure 119 is a spot film made during *Tussy's* BE, and Figure 120, a drawing. They show the barium column arrested in mid transverse colon by the intraluminal mass of intussuscepted ileum. This gradually withdraws into the right colon as the fluoroscopist watches it. The intussusception does not recur and *Tussy* makes an excellent recovery.

End of Case

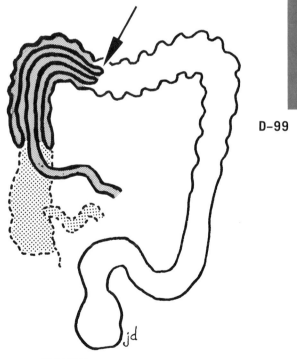

D-99

FIGURE 120. Intussusception

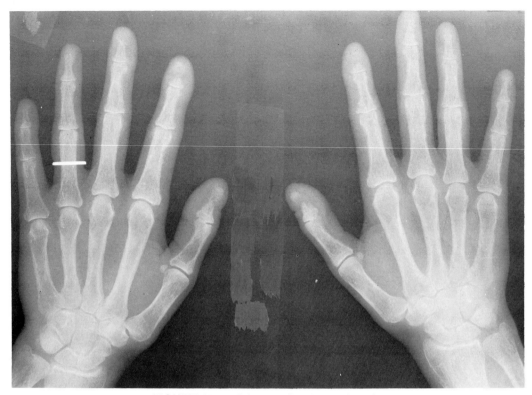

FIGURE 121. Adalena Cardoza's hands

Adalena Cardoza: *(Continued from page 73)* A 24-hour calcium excretion study indicates marked calciuria and the alkaline phosphatase is elevated. Nephrocalcinosis and a history of passing stones must make one think of the possibility of hyperparathyroidism. The laboratory values all tend to confirm this and hand films (Figs. 121 and 122) clinch the diagnosis. Note the marked subperiosteal resorption of bone along the margins of the phalanges. The patient agrees to an exploration of her neck and a parathyroid adenoma is resected. Unfortunately she had hyperparathyroidism for so long before it was discovered and corrected that her kidneys are irreparably damaged.

End of Case

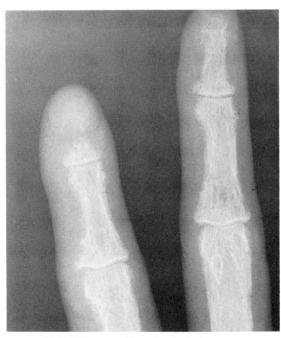

FIGURE 122. Detail of phalanges

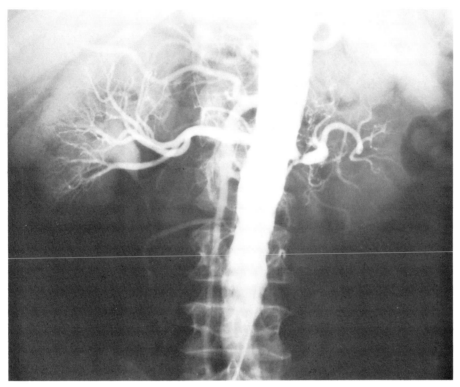

FIGURE 123. Rocco's aortogram

Rocco Malatesta: (*Continued from page 75*) In a hypertensive patient with a single small kidney demonstrating diminished function, you must consider a diagnosis of renal artery stenosis. Chronic atrophic pyelonephritis may also produce a single contracted kidney, but usually with more loss of renal cortex than is demonstrated on *Mr. Malatesta's* IVU.

The aortogram you requested (Fig. 123) clearly demonstrates a high-grade stenosis, classically located in the medial one-third of the left renal artery with post-stenotic dilatation. The stenosis is produced by an atherosclerotic plaque. Changes of atherosclerosis are also observed in the aorta, especially below the renal arteries where the lumen of this vessel is irregularly narrowed by multiple intimal plaques.

D–101

Renovascular hypertension may be treated medically or surgically. How would you treat *Mr. Malatesta*? Recent studies have shown that patients with renovascular hypertension given optimal medical therapy may do as well as those treated surgically. Because of *Mr. Malatesta's* history of previous myocardial infarct and his age, you elect to treat him medically. On a course of chlorothiazide and methyldopa his blood pressure drops to 140/100 and his headache disappears.

End of Case

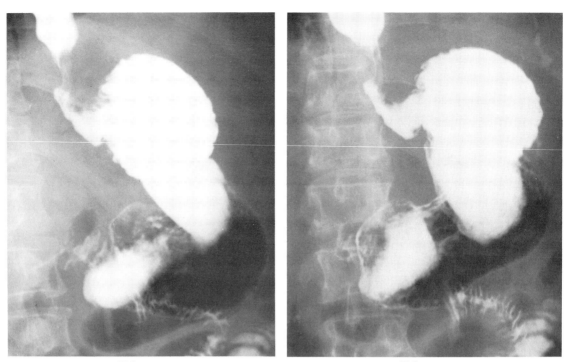

FIG. 124   FIG. 125

FIGURES 124 & 125.   Johnny Walker's stomach and esophagus

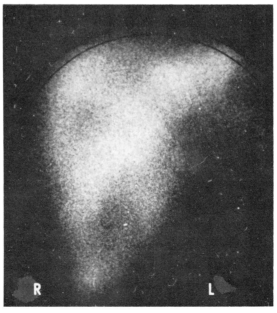

FIGURE 126.   Johnny's liver scan

Johnny Walker: *(Continued from page 80)* The history of anorexia and dysphagia directs your attention to the upper gastrointestinal tract. The presence of malignant disease has been confirmed by cytology. Suspecting an esophageal carcinoma or carcinoma of the stomach which has invaded the esophagus, you request an upper gastrointestinal series.

This study (Figs. 124 and 125) demonstrates a rigid constricting deformity of the distal esophagus and gastric cardia. The deformity is constant on all films and is diagnostic of carcinoma. The remainder of the stomach and duodenum and visualized loops of small bowel are normal.

The liver scan (Fig. 126) which you also requested depicts multiple areas of decreased uptake consistent with metastatic disease. Barium enema and IVU are normal.

Mr. Walker deteriorates in the hospital and suddenly expires. Post-mortem examination confirms the presence of gastric carcinoma which has infiltrated the lower esophagus and pancreas. There are metastases to regional lymph nodes, both pleurae, the pericardium, and the adrenal glands. Nearly the entire liver is replaced with metastases.

End of Case

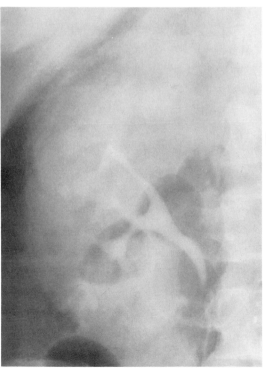

D–103

Luke Stein: *(Continued from page 63)* The most disturbing finding in this study is the persistent hump along the superior-lateral margin of the right kidney. On the detail film (Fig. 127) there appears to be an oval, 4 × 6 cm mass in the lateral portion of the upper pole of the right kidney which displaces the right upper pole calyces medially.

How will you confirm or rule out the presence of a right renal mass?

Continued Part E, page 118.

FIGURE 127. Luke's right kidney

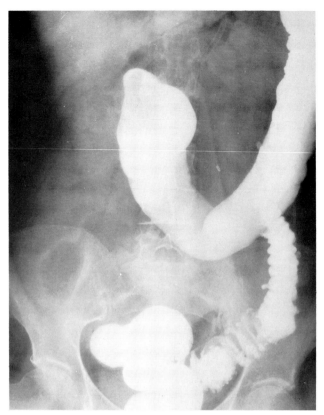

FIGURE 128. Lorraine Sheldon—AP film

Lorraine Sheldon: *(Continued from page 67)* Since the plain films of the abdomen indicate the probability of an obstructed colon and because emergency surgery is likely, you ask the radiologist to help you in pinpointing the exact location and cause of the obstruction by doing a barium enema. Here are AP and oblique films from that study (Figs. 128 and 129). The diagnosis?

Continued Part E, page 114.

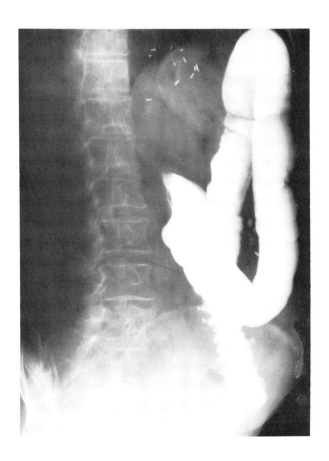

FIGURE 129. Oblique film

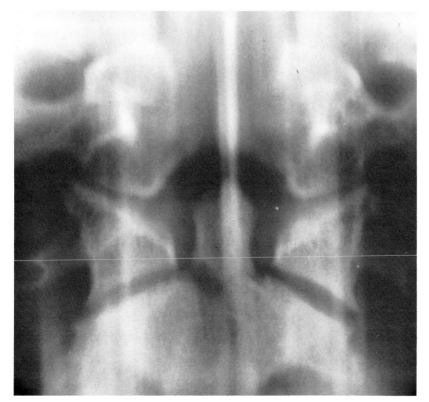

FIGURE 130. Tomogram of Clyde's odontoid

Clyde Lightfinger: (*Continued from page 59*) You can perform tomography of the cervical spine in the AP projection without any manipulation of the patient. It is an excellent method for visualizing the separate structures of the vertebrae. The cut taken at the level of the odontoid process shows a nondisplaced fracture of this structure at its base (Fig. 130).

Mr. Lightfinger is placed in a halo body cast which will both maintain cervical spine traction and allow him to be ambulatory. The pain and finger symptoms disappear. After 3 months the body cast is replaced with a soft collar for a fourth month. When this is removed, spine films show evidence of healing and the patient is completely asymptomatic.

Cervical spine fractures may be difficult to detect on plain radiographs. When you have a high degree of suspicion you should convey it to the radiology department so that special procedures such as tomography may be utilized.

End of Case

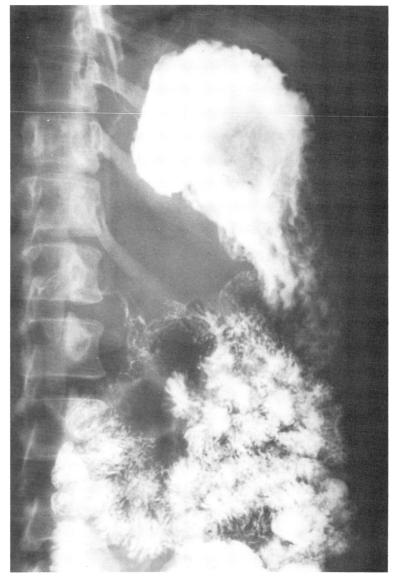

FIGURE 131. Cecily Mannerborn

Cecily Mannerborn: *(Continued from page 70)* An upper G.I. series is the most direct and least costly method for your purpose. Here is a film from that examination (Fig. 131). Well?

Continued Part E, page 128.

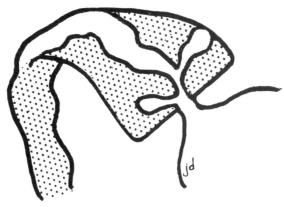

FIGURE 132. Diagram of Mr. Watling's severely deformed duodenal cap (in white) **superimposed on a normal cap for comparison** (dotted)

Carlton Watling: (*Continued from page 67*) The film from the upper G.I. series shows severe duodenal deformity from past ulcer disease. The maximum lumen at the most scarred portion of the duodenal cap measures only 2 mm (Fig. 132). By comparing this film with films which are available from 2 previous upper G.I. examinations, although the degree of scarring has increased, the radiologist feels that there is no new or active ulcer.

Obstruction, hemorrhage, and perforation are the three major complications of duodenal ulcer disease. *Watling's* recurrent obstruction is presumably due to a combination of scarring and edema brought on by his recent alcoholic and culinary binge. Because this is the third episode of obstruction, you advise *Watling* to have a subtotal gastrectomy and vagotomy.

End of Case

D–107

Penny Stone: (*Continued from page 61*) You are now left with a differential diagnosis between mesenteric adenitis and acute appendicitis. The former may mimic all the signs and symptoms of appendicitis, frequently being differentiated only at laparotomy. You take *Penny* to the operating room where you find evidence for acute appendicitis without a perforation. The serosal surface of the appendix is injected and covered with a fine white exudate. The appendix contains the expected appendolith.

A patient with acute unperforated appendicitis may have a completely normal abdominal film. If perforation has occurred, resulting in abscess formation, the abdominal film may show a right lower quadrant mass, localized small bowel ileus, scoliosis concave to the right, or a loss of the right psoas margin.

End of Case

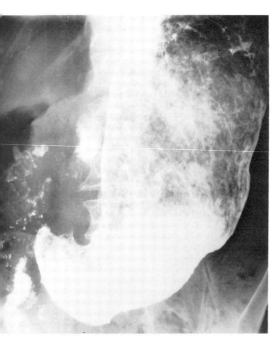

FIGURE 133. Captain Solent—food-, fluid- and barium-filled stomach

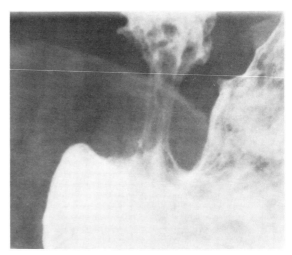

FIGURE 134. Detail of gastric antrum, constricted by tumor

Henry Mountjoy Solent: *(Continued from page 59)* Again it would be better to aspirate the gastric contents before doing a barium study, or if there seems to be a tremendous amount of fluid and food (and there is) to put the patient on gastric suction for 1 or 2 days. However, it is elected to give the patient several swallows of barium to define the degree of suspected gastric distention and to look for a gross cause. The large film (Fig. 133) shows a gigantic stomach filled with retained food and liquid, now mixed with the barium. A fluoroscopic spot film centered over the distal stomach (Fig. 134) shows rigid narrowing of the antrum, which would not distend more than 1 cm even with the full weight of gastric contents and barium against it.

Captain Solent has severe (but not complete) gastric outlet obstruction, which has undoubtedly been building up slowly for weeks. It is amazing how much fluid the stomach can contain in such a situation before the patient becomes aware of it, begins to vomit, and seeks attention.

Several days after decompression of this stomach by means of 36 hours of continuous suction, an exploratory laparotomy is performed and the distal antrum of the stomach is found to be diffusely infiltrated by carcinoma. Metastatic disease is already present in the liver, so only a palliative posterior gastroenterostomy is carried out.

End of Case

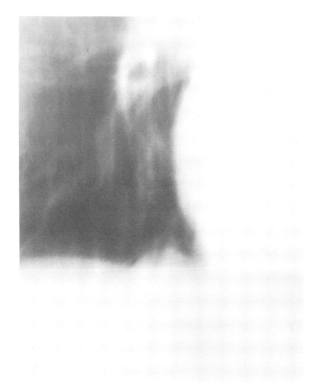

FIGURE 135. Laminogram of Ruby Reingold's right cardiophrenic angle

Ruby Hobson Reingold IV: *(Continued from page 79)* A laminographic cut might help and here it is (Fig. 135). The appearance of this mass strongly indicates a diaphragmatic origin. It is most unlikely that a tumor arising in the lung would have a convex upper margin and an inferior surface in such intimate contact with the diaphragm. Therefore, the mass may arise from the diaphragm or pleura, and, if so, leiomyoma, fibroma, neurofibroma, and lipoma are possibilities. Can you think of another way to further localize the mass? Please turn to *Part E, page 116.*

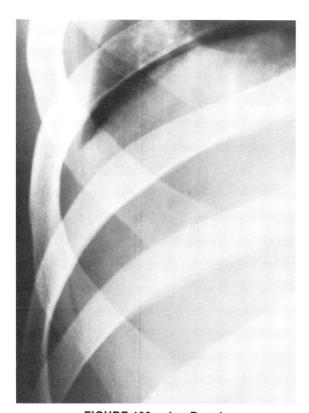

FIGURE 136. Jay Roach

Jay Roach: *(Continued from page 66)* You should always suspect possible liver injury in patients who have sustained right lower chest trauma. Stat liver function tests, amylase, and hematocrit are ordered. The LDH is elevated to 800, and the SGOT to 400. The hematocrit has dropped to 37 per cent. The amylase is normal.

You request a portable abdomen film which shows ileus, an elevated right hemidiaphragm and a previously not visualized right sixth rib fracture (detail film, Fig. 136). Also noted is a small right pleural fluid collection. What study will you ask for now?

Continued Part E, page 116.

D-109

FIGURE 137. Antonini—early phase of arteriogram

FIGURE 138. Detail, right flank

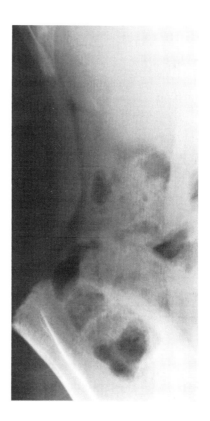

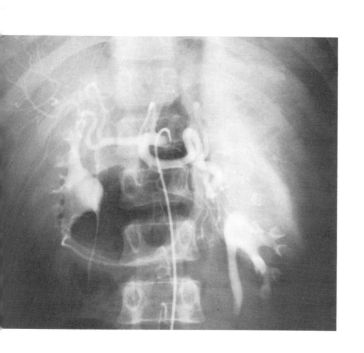

FIGURE 139. Late phase of arteriogram

Vittorio Antonini: *(Continued from page 75)* Put him on his right side for 10 minutes and then request another supine plain film with a light exposure (detail, Fig. 138). Note that the right flank stripe is normal (sharply defined) and not separated from the feces-and-air-filled right colon by a collection of free blood. The right flank is a better place to look for free blood than the left. A four-quadrant tap is negative.

You can also arrange for a celiac arteriogram to be done. Figures 137 and 139 (this patient's celiac studies) show a large nonopacified wedge between the splenic blush on the late film and the abdominal wall. There is also downward displacement of the left kidney and crowding medially of the splenic artery branches. These findings are diagnostic for a large subcapsular hematoma, and immediate surgery confirms your diagnosis. Premature discharge of patients with such hematomas has often resulted in death from sudden rupture and exsanguinating hemorrhage into the peritoneal space.

End of Case

Corey Bloat: *(Continued from page 82)* This inspiratory pressure drop is 15 mm Hg greater than the normal and is a sign of cardiac tamponade by a pericardial effusion. However, you should know that paradox may be absent, even with a large effusion, if the effusion is not tense.

All right, how will you confirm this clinical diagnosis? There are several ways of doing it. Any one of them may or may not be conclusive depending on the size of the effusion and the technical success of the procedure. How will you begin?

Please turn to *Part E, page 124.*

Maximilian Schock: *(Continued from page 60)* The family doctor is right. If this aneurysm is leaking, resection is probably necessary before it bursts. If it is not leaking, you can afford to temporize.

Mr. Schock is looking better, but his blood pressure is 90/60 and he is still having intermittent pain. You decide that you must operate. Will you follow the normal preoperative procedure and obtain an angiocardiogram to evaluate the coronary arteries and valves? Please turn to *Part E, page 115.*

PART E

PART E

Colette Vermilion: *(Continued from page 90)* Assuming that *Madame Vermilion* is in good physical condition and there are no medical contraindications to her having surgery, this polyp should be removed. It violates all the rules for safety: (1) the head is more than 1 cm in size; (2) the head is not round, but lobulated; and (3) the stalk is short and broad. In addition, the patient has rectal bleeding, presumably from this polyp—and a malignant polyp is more likely to bleed than a benign one. If, on the other hand, the head of the polyp in this patient had been 1 cm in size or less, if the head had been smooth and relatively round,

and if the stalk had been very long and thin, it might safely have been watched (Fig. 140). The chance of malignancy in this latter type of polyp is practically nil; it is a benign adenomatous polyp. However, the polyp in *Madame Vermilion's* colon is an ominous one and, although statistically most such polyps will also be benign, there is nothing about the appearance of this particular polyp to lend any reassurance that it is not malignant. The polyp is removed and it is a polypoid carcinoma. There are no signs of either local or distant metastases.

End of Case

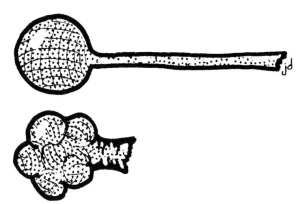

FIGURE 140. Diagrammatic contrast between characteristics usually associated with benign and malignant polyps (see text above)

Lorraine Sheldon: *(Continued from page 104)* There is incidental diverticulosis of the descending and sigmoid segments. The major finding on the films, however, confirms your suspicion of complete obstruction: the enema has stopped in the proximal transverse colon and the leading edge of the barium column defines a bulky tumor responsible for the obstruction.

The patient is taken to surgery. The right colon is found to be massively distended and the tumor in the proximal transverse colon can be palpated. A standard right colectomy is carried out, followed by an end-to-end ileotransverse colostomy. On microscopic examination the tumor is found to be an adenocarcinoma.

End of Case

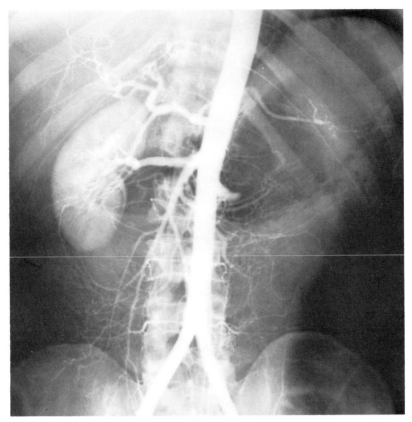

FIGURE 141. Chester's arteriogram

Chester Winston Wilcox: (*Continued from page 98*) Renal trauma suspects with a nonfunctioning kidney on an intravenous urogram must be evaluated for renal artery injury. You request an aortogram (Fig. 141) which demonstrates complete occlusion of the left renal artery.

Mr. Wilcox is promptly taken to the operating room for a left renal artery exploration. A thombosed segment of the left renal artery is discovered approximately 2 cm distal to the take-off of this vessel from the aorta. A 1.5 cm length of damaged renal artery is resected and an end-to-end anastomosis is performed. Postoperatively the patient does well and his left kidney begins to function.

Injuries to the renal parenchyma and renal artery in trauma patients are often associated with adjacent transverse process fractures, although *Mr. Wilcox* does not have one. It is postulated that his injury resulted from tension or stretching of the vessel.

End of Case

E–115

Maximilian Schock: (*Continued from page 111*) No. The pressure of the injection of contrast into the ventricle and the manipulation of an intracardiac catheter are too dangerous if this aneurysm is about to burst. Instead, *Mr. Shock* is taken to the operating room and the aneurysm is resected. The aneurysm was not, in fact, leaking. Please turn to *Part F, page 132,* for his postoperative film.

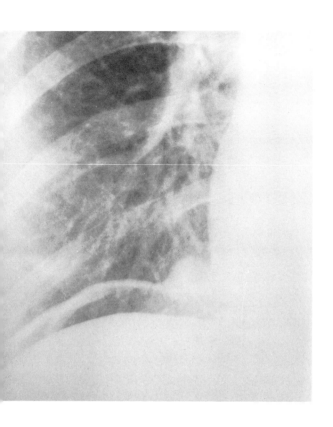

Ruby Hobson Reingold IV: *(Continued from page 109)* A diagnostic pneumoperitoneum is performed (Fig. 142). With air under the diaphragm it can now be seen that this mass extends both above and below the diaphragm, with sloping margins at the diaphragm and a convex upper surface. This makes diaphragmatic origin most likely and excludes a lesion arising in the lung itself or in an abdominal organ and projecting into the thorax. The information thus gained will be invaluable in planning the surgical approach. The surgeon finds a benign fibroma of the diaphragm. Look at the postoperative film in *Part F, page 134.*

FIGURE 142. Ruby Hobson Reingold IV

Jay Roach: *(Continued from page 109)* Now you have strong evidence for a hepatic injury and you request a liver scan (Fig. 143). It shows a discrete defect in the dome of the right lobe of the liver compatible with a subcapsular hematoma. Which study will confirm this diagnosis?

Continued Part F, page 136.

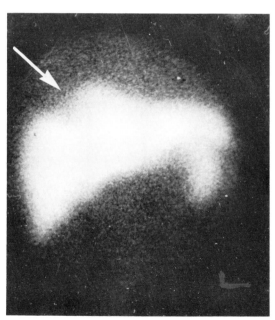

FIGURE 143. Jay's liver scan

Ernest Waters: *(Continued from page 87)* His symptoms are consistent with both uremia and metastatic disease. Stat BUN and creatinine levels are normal. An intravenous urogram demonstrates normal functioning kidneys and an ileal loop. A bone series which includes the lumbar spine is unremarkable, with no evidence of metastases. What do you see on *Mr. Waters'* chest film and liver scan in *Part F, page 138?*

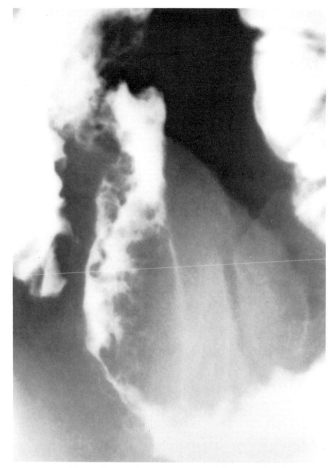

FIGURE 144. Spot film of Miss Feld's terminal ileum

Hannah Feld: *(Continued from page 96)*
The terminal ileum is abnormal (Fig. 144, a detail film). The last 6 inches show irregular narrowing and an abnormal "cobblestone" appearance of the mucosa due to criss-crossing ulcers and fissures that define islands of hyperplastic mucosa. There is also slight proximal dilatation of the ileum, and there is an increase in soft tissue density on either side of the terminal ileum due to surrounding inflammatory induration. It displaces adjacent small bowel loops to the left. The slightly dilated distal small bowel and the inflammatory "mass" could both be at least suspected on the initial plain film.

These x-ray findings are characteristic of terminal ileitis (regional ileitis or granulomatous ileitis), a disease which affects young adults, not infrequently Jewish, and presents as a febrile illness with cramps and either diarrhea or constipation. Gross bleeding is rare and there is a significant incidence of concomitant or future involvement of the colon by the same process. In fact, this patient, who initially does well on Azulfidine and a low roughage diet, returns 9 months later with involvement of the cecum and ascending colon.

End of Case

E-117

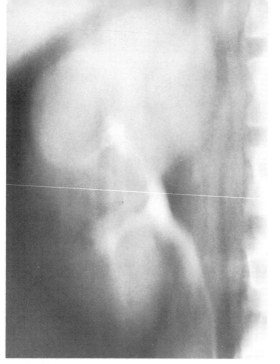

FIGURE 145. Luke's nephrotomogram

Luke Stein: *(Continued from page 103)* For further evaluation of the right kidney you request intravenous nephrotomography. In this procedure, laminographic cuts of the kidneys are taken while the patient is concurrently receiving an intravenous infusion of contrast medium. The films obtained visualize the renal parenchyma better than the early films of the standard IVU.

The cut reproduced here (Fig. 145) confirms the suspected right renal mass. It appears to have a thick oval rim. How will you differentiate a renal cyst from a renal tumor?

Continued Part F, page 137.

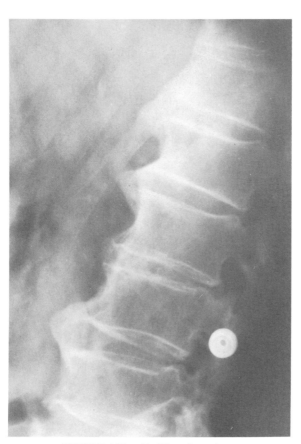

FIGURE 146. Dollface's spine

Dollface Davenport: *(Continued from page 87)* The gallbladder is not visualized on the first or second dose of contrast medium. Here is a lateral view of the lumbar spine (Fig. 146).

The slight narrowing of the vertebral interspaces and "lipping" of osteophytes around the margins of the vertebrae are changes of osteoarthritis. There is no bone destruction, obliteration of interspaces, or soft tissue mass as might be expected with osteomyelitis.

What about that gallbladder? The failure to concentrate the contrast is worrisome, but there are no symptoms of gallbladder inflammation and the stool cultures are negative for salmonella, making it highly unlikely that the gallbladder is a reservoir of infection. You must look elsewhere.

How much does the persistent recovery of the organism from the blood cultures mean to you? Can you think of any other diagnostic possibilities? Please turn to *Part F, page 135.*

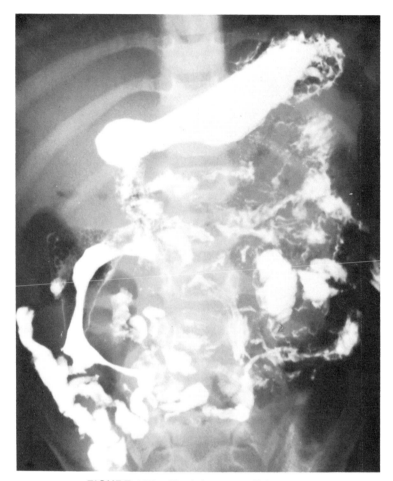

FIGURE 147. Kevin's upper G.I. series

Kevin Somers: *(Continued from page 89)* Here are the upper G.I. series and a small bowel follow-through. The stomach and duodenum are probably normal, but most of the small bowel is not. Bowel loops do not sit closely together as they usually do, and several loops are so stretched and distorted that the mucosal folds are effaced. There is not one mass, but multiple masses throughout the mesentery, so that the small intestine has lost its pliability. Look at that C-shaped loop of ileum on the right. Now glance back at the plain film and IVP. That fixed loop does not contract; it was visible on both previous studies.

Well, what sort of tumor is this spreading throughout the mesentery, causing an anemia and unusual masses? Please turn to *Part F, page 133,* for the chest film which will confirm your diagnosis.

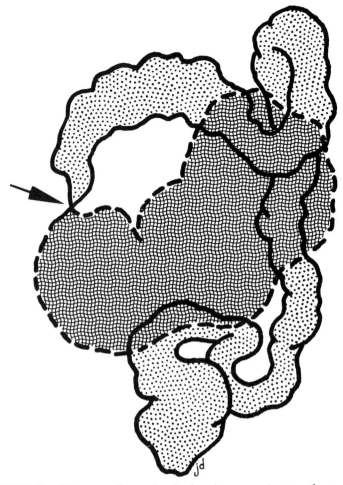

FIGURE 148. **Diagram of cecal volvulus** (arrow points to the twist)

Pierre Claude Tordu: *(Continued from page 94)* The pre- and post-evacuation films from the barium enema show that barium has outlined normal colon up to a point just proximal to the hepatic flexure. No further passage of barium into the right colon or cecum has occurred. The large gas- and feces-filled structure is still seen occupying most of the left side of the abdomen.

This picture is just about classic for a full-blown cecal volvulus. A cecal volvulus may occur, usually presenting as an acute large bowel obstruction, in patients who have a very mobile cecum. This mobility is due to incomplete rotation of the colon, or to failure of fixation of the ascending colon after proper rota-

tion. These rotation events are normally completed successfully in the 12th fetal week.

Volvulus most often occurs in males in mid or late life. If the mobile cecum should become twisted on itself, as it did in *Monsieur Tordu's* case, it then gradually distends, with gas passing into it from normal small bowel. The distention becomes so great that the cecum moves out of its usual position in the right lower abdomen and is forced into the mid or left abdomen. The plain film of the abdomen will show the hugely dilated air shadow of the cecum in an unexpected position. There is almost always a fair amount of gas in the small bowel, whereas the colon distal to the twist is empty. A barium enema will confirm the suspected diagnosis by revealing a normal distal colon up to the point of twist. The column of barium frequently ends abruptly with a funnel-shaped configuration that represents the actual point of twist. The air-distended cecum, and often a portion of the ascending colon, will be seen to occupy an abnormal position in the mid or left abdomen (Fig. 148). You schedule the patient for surgery. A right colectomy is performed.

End of Case

Lucy Rouge: *(Continued from page 89) Mrs. Rouge* is transferred to the surgical service, where she has the benefit of another medical student work-up. On taking the history the student elicits that approximately 2 weeks prior to the onset of cough, *Lucy* had had a tooth extracted and the gum had been packed. On awakening the next morning, she found the pack gone and assumed that she had swallowed it. The surgeons elect a trial of antibacterial and anti-tuberculous chemotherapy. However, serial chest films over the next 2 weeks show no improvement. At operation there is no tumor present. There is a thick-walled abscess approximately 2 cm in diameter distal to the fragment of packing in the bronchus. *Mrs. Rouge* recovers and goes back to her cook books and poetry. She sent us her favorite recipe. Here it is:

Lucy's Paté

If you would know how to impress your friends
    Then learn to make this luscious canapé,
And I assure you there's no butter way,
    If you've offended them, to make amends!
Butter, four sticks (use one, reserve the rest)
    Softened; two cups of chicken livers, fine;
Brown shallots, chopped and sautéed, nine;
    A cup of cognac, better than the best!

Black truffles, two; one teaspoon each of salt
    And pepper will complete the list you need.
Sauté the livers (not too much, take heed!),
    Add brandy, flame. Stand back! It's not my fault
If, careless, you have singed your hair!
    Now blend, and just before you mold and chill,
Work in those last three sticks of butter, still,
    ——And say it isn't simple if you dare!

End of Case

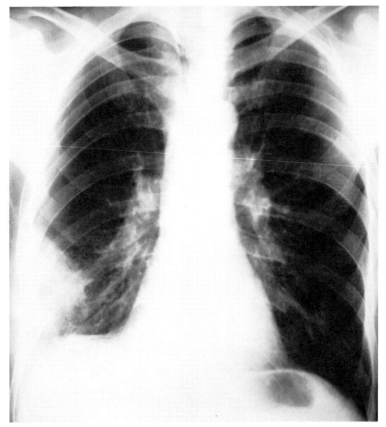

FIGURE 149. Jack's second post-op chest film

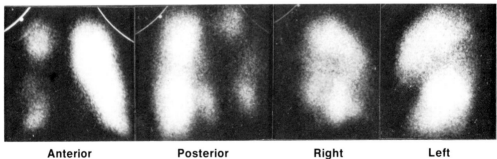

Anterior   Posterior   Right   Left

FIGURE 150.   Jack's lung scan

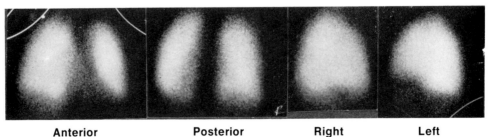

Anterior   Posterior   Right   Left

FIGURE 151.   A normal scan

Jack Eveready: *(Continued from page 88)* Two days later, *Mr. Eveready* has a second episode of poorly localized chest pain. This time he is short of breath, but his physical examination is unchanged. Here are his chest film (Fig. 149) and lung scan (Fig. 150), and a normal scan for comparison (Fig. 151).

The patchy infiltrate has become a well-defined, wedge-shaped, pleural-based density. The lateral film showed this density to be posterior. Comparing the chest x-ray with the lung scan, you can see diminished activity in several areas other than the right lower lobe. This is a positive scan.

If the only area of decreased activity were in the region of the infiltrate, this scan would not help you, since capillary perfusion may be decreased in many infiltrates including pneumonia. The areas of diminished activity that are not associated with infiltrates are presumably caused by emboli that have reduced the segmental blood supply without actually causing a lung infarction.

There isn't really any point in doing a pulmonary arteriogram at this time because the diagnosis has been firmly established. *Jack* is given anticoagulants and recovers uneventfully.

End of Case

Alfred Stevens: *(Continued from page 92)* No. Even though the liver and spleen appear to be normal, there may be microscopic involvement of these organs. The spleen is so commonly involved when the mediastinum is diseased that you are obliged to examine it. If the lymphangiogram were equivocal, the laparotomy would also give you a chance to remove and examine any suspicious nodes. The spleen is normal at laparotomy.

Here is a post-irradiation chest film (Fig. 152) showing shrinkage of the mass and some paramediastinal fibrosis.

Mr. Stevens is asymptomatic and apparently cured 5 years after the diagnosis was made.

This case is a typical example of the way in which lymphoma should be evaluated. The mode of treatment and prognosis depend upon an exact knowledge of the extent of the disease at the time of diagnosis.

End of Case

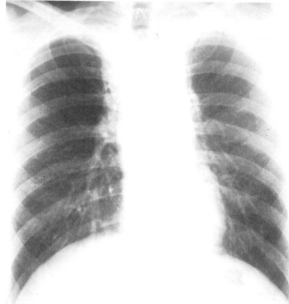

E–123

FIGURE 152. Stevens' post-irradiation chest film

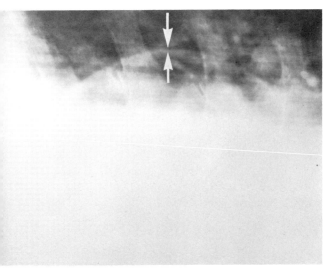

FIGURE 153. Normal CO$_2$ study

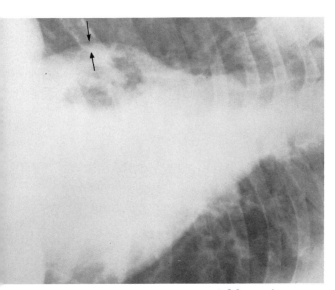

FIGURE 154. Bloat—abnormal CO$_2$ study

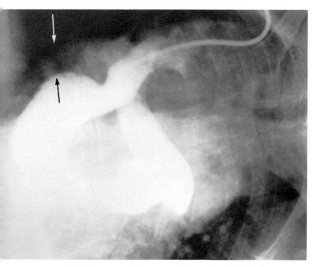

FIGURE 155. Abnormal contrast study

Corey Bloat: *(Continued from page 111)* At cardiac fluoroscopy the radiologist may see very little cardiac motion or pulsation. This is not diagnostic, since a flabby myocardium may also show little pulsation. Sometimes, however, you can see a crescent of epicardial fat at the cardiac apex pulsating in a bag of water-density pericardial fluid. If you do, the diagnosis is confirmed.

The most frequently discussed method is to infuse sterile CO$_2$ or, nowadays, contrast material through a central venous catheter while the patient is positioned with his left side down. The CO$_2$ will be trapped in the right atrium, showing a wall only 2 or 3 mm in thickness. An effusion will produce an apparent thickening of this wall (Figs. 153, 154, and 155.)

Incidentally, Figure 153 shows you what to do when you suspect that a patient has an air embolus. Patients with lacerated neck veins or disconnected CVP lines may suck air into the right heart. If this air is allowed to lodge in the right ventricular outflow tract, the blood flow to the lungs will be stopped and the patient will have a "mill wheel" murmur followed by cardiorespiratory arrest. Patients suspected of air embolism should therefore be immediately positioned with the left side down.

Part F shows you 2 more ways to show this rim of fluid around the heart. These methods are especially easy on the patient and, incidentally, would be useful in a patient who is allergic to contrast media. Can you anticipate what they are? Please turn to *Part F, page 134.*

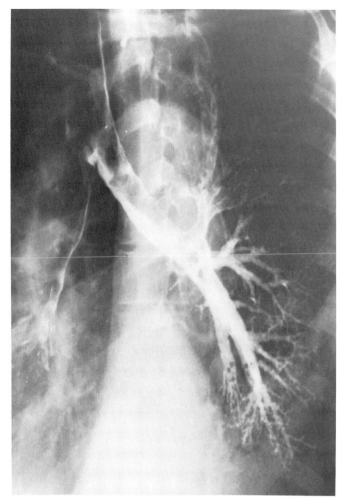

FIGURE 156. Sgt. Kent's bronchogram

Amanda Kent *(Continued from page 86)* You admit *Sergeant Kent* to the Base Hospital. This can no longer be an atypical pneumonia. Tuberculosis is still a possibility, but her skin test is negative. Pneumonias distal to endobronchial lesions may clear slowly but these are usually bacterial infections with more symptoms and more damage to the lung. The air bronchograms speak against bronchial obstruction.

In an attempt to get a good look at the lower lobe and a good sputum sample, you perform bronchoscopy. No bronchial lesion is seen. The next day you obtain a bronchogram. Here is the left lower lobe bronchogram (Fig. 156).

The bronchi in the area of the infiltrate are narrowed and irregular. There may be some slight loss of volume, since the terminal bronchi do not spread out but are bunched together. Turn to *Part F, page 139*, for the diagnosis.

E–125

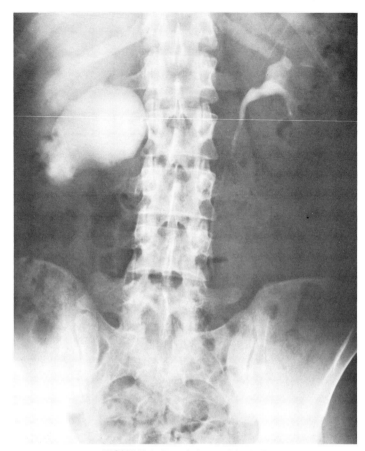

FIGURE 157.   Adumreb's IVP

Dr. Notlimah Adumreb: *(Continued from page 94)* Remembering that the right kidney has appeared somewhat larger than normal on previous films, you decide to wait several days for the barium to clear the entire G.I. tract and then, finally, to do an intravenous pyelogram. This is the 30 minute film (Fig. 157), and the problem is solved. *Dr. Adumreb* has a moderately severe right hydronephrosis. The upper surface of the dilated renal pelvis corresponds exactly to the original point of obstruction in the duodenum (Fig. 158). Presumably, this pelvis was even larger at the time it caused acute obstruction during the long flight back to this country. At surgery, an anomalous right renal artery is found crossing anterior to the ureteropelvic junction and causing near complete obstruction to outflow of urine. This artery supplies the lower pole of the right kidney.

End of Case

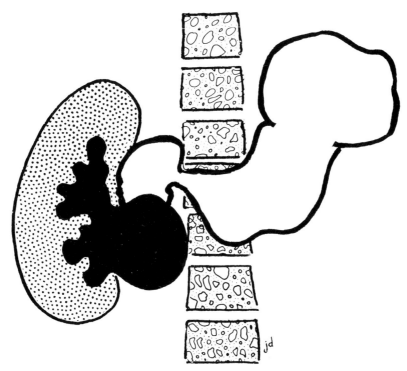

FIGURE 158.   How the obstruction occurred

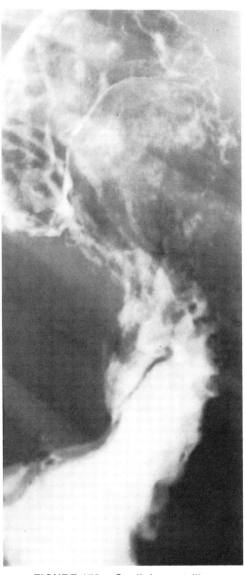

FIGURE 159. Cecily's spot film

Cecily Mannerborn *(Continued from page 106)* The upper G.I. series shows a filling defect which represents a mass either arising from the posterior wall of the gastric fundus or arising outside of the stomach, indenting it from behind, and better visualized on this fluoroscopic spot film (Fig. 159).

Putting it all together, you remember that among the complications of chronic pancreatitis are diabetes and pseudocyst of the pancreas. Left-sided pleural effusion may be seen in patients with pancreatitis and its persistence after an acute attack may be a clue to the presence of a pseudocyst of the pancreas.

You next perform gastroscopy and find that the "gastric mass" can be identified, but it appears to be extrinsic to the stomach. For a still more refined evaluation, you now request a celiac arteriogram, which shows depression of the splenic artery with splaying of multiple normal splenic branches around a large avascular mass (Figs. 160 and 161).

At surgery, a large pseudocyst arising from the tail of the pancreas is found. The cyst extends into the hilum of the spleen and is also in continuity with the inferior surface of the diaphragm and the posterior wall of the stomach. The pancreas itself appears to be involved by chronic pancreatitis, and there are multiple small areas of fat necrosis.

End of Case

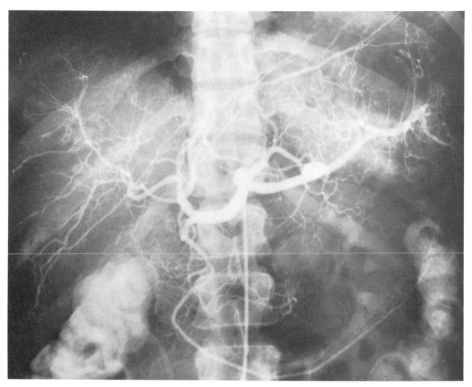

FIGURE 160.   Cecily's celiac arteriogram

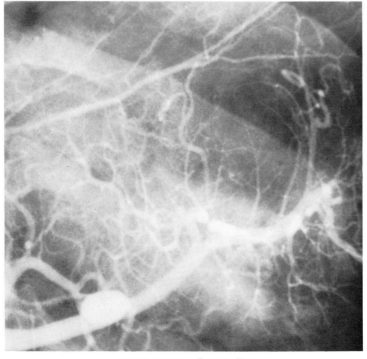

FIGURE 161.   Detail film

PART F

PART F

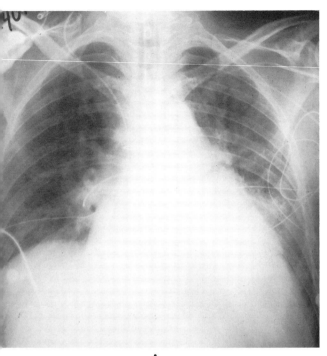

A

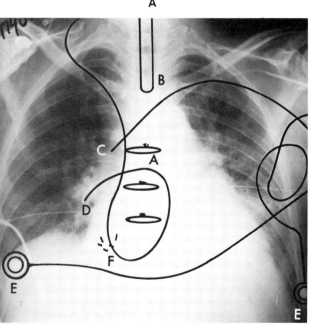

B

FIGURE 162A & B. Mr. Schock's post-op chest

Maximilian Schock: *(Continued from page 115)* The aneurysm has been resected. What do you make of the heart and pulmonary vasculature (Fig. 162)? This is a portable film. The heart is now almost normal in size and shape. The pulmonary vasculature is distended and there are small perihilar infiltrates. *Mr. Schock* is in congestive heart failure with some pulmonary edema. Can you identify the various tubes, catheters, and wires that you see here?

The heart was approached by splitting the sternum. Those are wire sutures in the sternum (*A*). The endotracheal tube is visible with its tip safely proximal to the carina (*B*). An intravenous catheter extends from the left arm to the superior vena cava to measure the central venous pressure (*C*). A similar softer catheter from the right external jugular vein passes through the right atrium and ventricle into a pulmonary artery where it is possible to measure the pulmonary wedge pressure (*D*). This gives a better assessment of left ventricular function than does the central venous pressure. Overlying the chest are monitor leads (*E*), but there are also small wires and clips which are barely visible on this film and which project over the right atrium and ventricle (*F*). These are silver wires embedded in the heart which can be used to pace the heart in an emergency. When the patient recovers, these are cut off at skin level.

Here are the final PA and lateral films of the new *Mr. Schock!* (Figs. 163 and 164). Except for the remaining sutures and pacing wire remnants, it is almost a normal heart.

End of Case

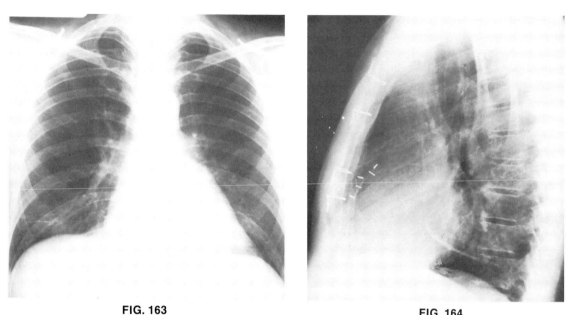

FIG. 163

FIG. 164

FIGURES 163 & 164.   The new Mr. Schock

Kevin Somers: *(Continued from page 119)* This portable chest film obtained late in *Kevin's* illness shows the mediastinum widened by mediastinal and paratracheal lymph nodes. *Kevin* has widespread lymphocytic lymphoma.

End of Case

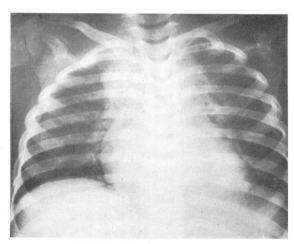

FIGURE 165.   Kevin Somers

F–133

Ruby Hobson Reingold IV: *(Continued from page 116)* This and other postoperative films show persistent elevation of the right hemidiaphragm. At surgery the tumor was near the right phrenic nerve and the surgeon was unable to remove it without injuring the nerve.

End of Case

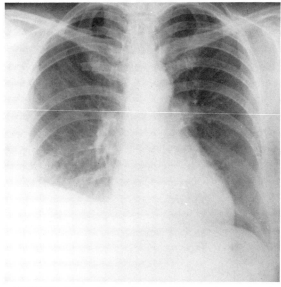

FIGURE 166. Ruby Reingold's post-op chest

Corey Bloat: *(Continued from page 124)* This is an isotopic scan in which the blood pools of the cardiac chambers, the lungs, and the liver are filled with radioactive isotope, in this case technetium-99. The lucent area outlining the heart is the pericardial effusion. (The isotope could be made to remain in the lung and liver for several hours, if necessary, by binding it to iron hydroxide and to sulfur colloid, respectively.)

Ultrasound can also be used, since the sound waves will be reflected off both the pericardium and epicardium, which will be separated from each other by the effusion. This method is so simple and nonhazardous that it may well become the method of choice in the future.

End of Case

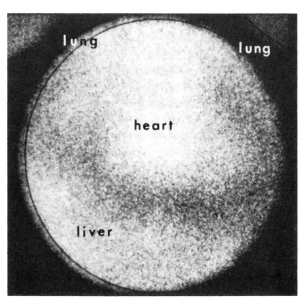

FIGURE 167. Scan of a pericardial effusion—dark area around heart is effusion

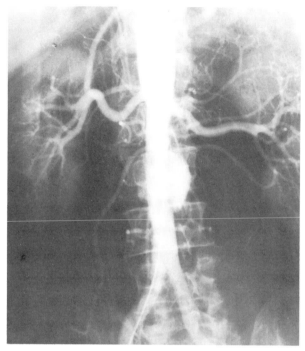

FIGURE 168. Dollface Davenport's aortogram

Dollface Davenport: *(Continued from page 118)* Could a mycotic aneurysm be the source? You re-examine *Dollface* but hear no murmurs and feel no mass. He has lost another 15 lbs while in the hospital under treatment. You request an aortogram (Fig. 168).

That is the source: a mycotic aneurysm of the aorta just below the renal arteries! If you thought of it, you should congratulate yourself because only one house officer and the infectious disease consultant included it in their differential.

Once the aneurysm is resected, the salmonella responds to chloramphenicol and *Dollface* recovers uneventfully.

Fevers of unknown origin are a very difficult problem. They have often been partially treated before you see them and have often proved a dilemma for another physician. Occasionally a diagnostic laparotomy is needed to make the diagnosis, and even that drastic procedure may be fruitless.

Complicated as this case is, it is representative of the step-by-step analysis necessary to unravel these challenging medical mysteries.

End of Case **F-135**

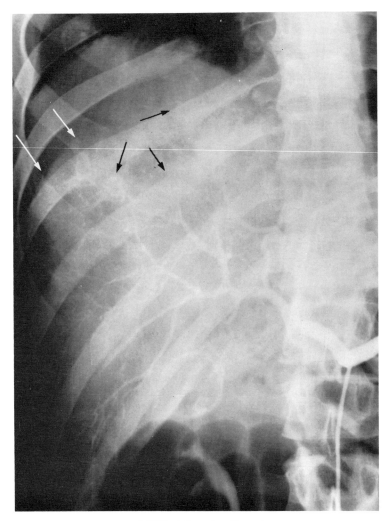

FIGURE 169. Jay Roach

Jay Roach: *(Continued from page 116)* The hepatic arteriogram (Fig. 169) clearly outlines the subcapsular hematoma by a separation of the vascularized liver parenchyma (white arrows) from the right hemidiaphragm and right lateral rib cage. The source of bleeding appears to be a laceration (black arrows) which is seen as a defect in the vascularized parenchyma of the dome of the right lobe.

Presumably *Mr. Roach* entered the hospital with a small hepatic laceration related to the right rib fracture. The laceration was not clinically suspected at that time, but apparently began to bleed, producing a subcapsular hematoma once anticoagulants had been administered. The rib fracture was not seen on the admission films. This is not surprising, since small rib fractures may be extremely difficult to visualize and appropriate rib films were not taken.

Mr. Roach's anticoagulant therapy is stopped. He is taken to the operating room where the hematoma is evacuated and the hepatic laceration is repaired. Postoperatively he makes an uneventful recovery.

End of Case

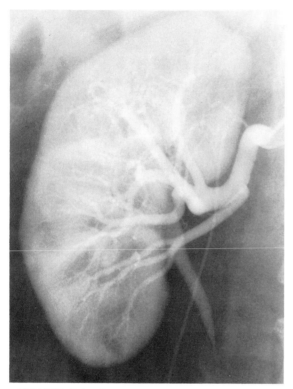

FIGURE 170. Luke Stein's renal arteriogram

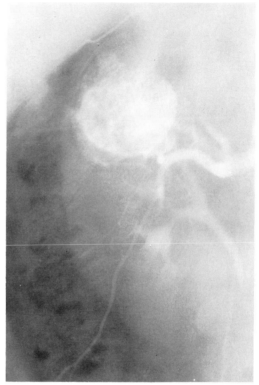

FIGURE 171. Arteriogram after epinephrine

Luke Stein: *(Continued from page 118)* You request a selective renal arteriogram (Fig. 170) which demonstrates a diffuse nephrogram throughout the right kidney. The area of the mass is vascular although some of the vessels appear abnormal. There is no evidence of a renal cyst. Cysts contain fluid and are avascular. They are characterized angiographically by round, well-circumscribed areas of absent nephrogram.

While the right renal artery catheter is still in place, the radiologist does an "epinephrine run." Prior to a second injection of contrast, he administers a small volume of a dilute epinephrine solution through the catheter. This drug will produce vasoconstriction in the normal renal vessels but no response in tumor vessels. The vessels in the mass (Fig. 171) do not constrict, and you can be certain that this mass is a tumor.

Dr. Stein is scheduled for a right nephrectomy. A small renal cell carcinoma without any evidence of metastatic disease is found.

It is indeed fortunate when an asymptomatic cancer is diagnosed early as a result of a fortuitous incident.

End of Case

F-137

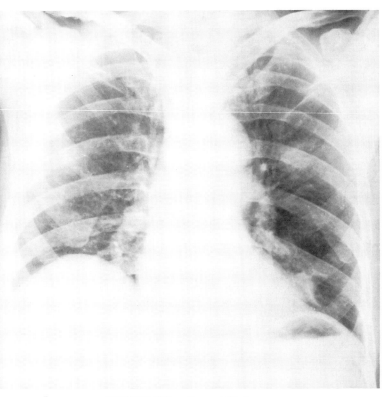

FIGURE 172. Ernest Waters

Ernest Waters: *(Continued from page 116)* His chest film (Fig. 172) shows several soft tissue pulmonary densities. Multiple areas of diminished uptake are seen in the liver scan (Fig. 173). Both studies are consistent with metastatic disease.

You request a bone scan for further evaluation of the lumbar spine; this study is occasionally positive in patients with normal plain films. *Mr. Waters* may derive some symptomatic relief from palliative radiotherapy to his spine if metastases are the cause of his pain, but before the scan is performed, the patient suddenly expires, and permission for autopsy is denied.

End of Case

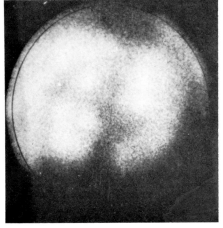

FIGURE 173. Ernest Waters' liver scan

Amanda Kent: *(Continued from page 125)* The bronchoscopy is normal; those irregular terminal bronchi are too distal to be visualized with a bronchoscope. One of 2 cytologic smears shows "one clump of small suspicious cells." At thoracotomy, an alveolar cell carcinoma is discovered. The right effusion probably reflects metastases even though normal pleural fluid is obtained when it is tapped.

Alveolar cell carcinomas, which are thought to arise from the epithelium of the terminal or respiratory bronchioles, make up from 3 to 15 per cent of lung cancers. This history, typical for mycoplasma pneumonia, is also classic for this tumor, especially when the infiltrate persists for several weeks. This tumor may also present as one or more nodules in the lung, but a pneumonic presentation is not uncommon.

End of Case

F–139